Å. Hjalmarson, W.J. Remme (Eds.)

Sinus node inhibitors

A new concept in angina pectoris

Steinkopff Verlag Darmstadt
Springer-Verlag New York

The Editors:
Prof. Å. Hjalmarson
Professor of Cardiology
Gothenburg University
Wallenberg Laboratory for
Cardiovascular Research
Sahlgren's Hospital
S-41345 Gothenburg

Dr. W.J. Remme
STICARES
Cardiovascular Research Foundation
Valkeniersweg 79
NL-3075 AZ Rotterdam

Die Deutsche Bibliothek – CIP-Einheitsaufnahme

Sinus node inhibitors : a new concept in angina pectoris / Å. Hjalmarson ; W. Remme (ed.). – Darmstadt : Steinkopff ; New York : Springer, 1991
ISBN-13:978-3-7985-0861-3 e-ISBN-13:978-3-642-72458-9
DOI: 10.1007/978-3-642-72458-9

NE: Hjalmarson, Åke [Hrsg.]

Medical Editorial: Sabine Müller – English Editor: James C. Willis –
Production: Heinz J. Schäfer

Type-setting: Mitterweger Werksatz, Plankstadt

Printed on acid-free paper

Foreword

Although surgical and catheter-based revascularization techniques have substantially improved today's therapeutic potential in ischemic heart disease, in the majority of patients treatment will be conservative for a number of reasons, the cost-effectiveness of non-pharmacological approaches being of major importance. During the last two decades, drug development for ischemic heart disease has been impressive and many new compounds have been added to our therapeutic armamentarium. Nevertheless, where mode of action is concerned, it is interesting to note that, despite all these efforts, we are still confined to three categories of drugs. Antithrombotics and platelet-active agents aside, these concern nitrates, betablocking drugs and calcium antagonists, agents which reduce ischemia by diminishing cardiac work or wall stress, thereby affecting myocardial oxygen demand and/or by improving coronary blood flow. Alone or in combination, these agents have proved to be efficacious in the treatment of angina pectoris or other symptoms of ischemic heart disease in a number of patients, but certainly not in all. Moreover, as side-effects are often a problem with current antianginal compounds, the physician may find himself restricted in his therapeutic capabilities and in need of new and, preferably, alternative forms of pharmacological treatment.

This has been recognized by pharmaceutical companies and has led to several interesting new developments. Although often in their initial stages, novel, but promising concepts in antiischemic pharmacological therapy include calmodulin antagonists, potassium channel modulators, intracellular-acting antioxidants, and agents which have direct myocardial metabolic effects, such as carnitine derivatives. Moreover, for certain conditions, modulation of ischemia-induced neurohumoral activation by converting-enzyme inhibitors may be of therapeutic value.

A different novel concept in antiischemic therapy, sinus node inhibition, is addressed in this volume. Reduction of heart rate as a mechanism to limit myocardial oxygen demand is, of course, not a new concept, this being one of the major effects of betablocking drugs and certain calcium antagonists. However, specific slowing of heart rhythm through a selective reduction of the spontaneous diastolic depolarization rate of the sinus node without concomitant effects on the heart is certainly a novel approach. Sinus node inhibitors (also referred to as "specific bradycardic agents") which have been developed up to now include the clonidine-derivative alinidine, falipamil – a modification of verapamil – and the benzazepinone derivative ULFS 49 CL. It is the latter which, through its specificity, appears to be the agent of choice in this class.

Consequently, this volume mainly concerns animal and clinical research with ULFS 49 CL. In both, the potential of the drug to limit or prevent myocardial ischemia through a modulating effect on heart rate during exercise without other apparent activities is clearly demonstrated. It is striking that, in the clinical studies presented in this volume, the antiischemic properties of ULFS 49 CL appear rather pronounced in relation to the moderate reductions in heart rate, both at rest and during exercise. This suggests that different, as yet unknown, mechanisms of action may still be present.

Moreover, it indicates that this challenging and promising new concept in the treatment of myocardial ischemia needs to be investigated further. Besides mechanisms of action, the place of ULFS 49 CL in the treatment of myocardial ischemia as first-line therapy or added to currently available medication should be explored, as well as its potential usefulness in other areas of cardiovascular medicine.

W. J. Remme

Contents

Reduction of heart rate – Really a new concept in treating angina pectoris?

Å. Hjalmarson

Division of Cardiology, Department of Medicine I, and Wallenberg Laboratory, University of Göteborg, Sahlgren's Hospital Göteborg, Sweden

Summary

Myocardial ischemia causing chest pain in patients with angina pectoris is due to an imbalance between coronary blood flow and myocardial metabolic demand. Heart rate is a major determinant of oxygen consumption and metabolic demand, and drugs known to reduce heart rate, such as β-blockers and some calcium blockers have well established effects in patients with angina pectoris. In addition to its importance as a determinant of oxygen consumption, heart rate is also an independent predictor, both of risk of developing acute myocardial infarction as well as a predictor for later complications including death. Increased heart rate can be due to either increased sympathetic activity and/or reduced parasympathetic activity. Psychosocial stress, an important risk factor for development of coronary artery disease, is characterized by an increase in heart rate and systolic blood pressure. β-blockers and calcium blockers are well established in the therapy of ischemic heart disease, and β-blockers are also known to reduce and prevent infarct development and mortality after myocardial infarction. It seems reasonable to believe that new drugs with specific effects on heart rate, without any influence on contractility, could be useful in the therapy of patients with ischemic heart disease, with symptoms of angina pectoris, as well as with supraventricular tachycardia and congestive heart failure.

Introduction

The treatment of patients with angina pectoris and other symptoms of ischemic heart disease has changed markedly over the last two decades. New therapies have been introduced and become widely accepted. These include various medications such as antiischemics (β-blockers, calcium channel blockers, nitrates), antiplatelets (salicylic acid, dihydropyridamole), and antithrombotics (salicylic acid, anticoagulants), and mechanical revascularizations (CABG, PTCA, atherectomy). The treatments are aimed at either a reduction of heart work/metabolic demand and/or improvement of coronary blood flow. All antiischemic drugs reduce heart work more or less markedly by affecting heart rate, pressure development and ventricular wall stress. Heart rate is the most important determinant of oxygen consumption and heart work and a prevention of unwanted stress-induced increase of heart rate is therefore obvious (4, 20).

β-blockers and some calcium channel blockers elicit their major antiischemic effects through a control of heart rate (3, 23). The concept of reducing heart rate in the treatment of patients with angina pectoris is well established and not new. The introduction of a new class of sinus node inhibitors which reduce heart rate without influencing contractility offers, however, new treatment possibilities. Patients with adverse reactions to β-blockers and calcium channel blockers may benefit especially, and in others heart rate reduction can be further potentiated by a combined use of new and old drugs. The present work discusses the heart rate in angina pectoris and in ischemic heart disease, and also the potential role of the new class of sinus node inhibitors.

Pathology of angina pectoris

The majority of patients with angina pectoris has the stable type where chest pain is induced by physical exercise or mental stress (4, 20). An increase in sympathetic activity causes elevation of heart rate and systolic blood pressure. These major determinants of cardiac oxygen consumption raise the metabolic demand and should be met by an increase in coronary blood supply. A restricted flow due to a critical coronary artery stenosis will result in myocardial ischemia due to an imbalance between metabolic demand and coronary flow. During the last 10 years, other mechanisms behind the ischemic attack have been put forward which may modify the ischemic response to physical or mental stress. The term "mixed type of angina pectoris" is used to explain why, for example, cold and windy weather makes effort angina worse, and being induced at a lower workload (19). A change in coronary artery vasomotor tone and/or thrombocyte aggregation are most likely involved (21, 30). A true vasospasm is known to cause chest pain at rest or at low work load in a smaller subset of patients. A defect coronary artery autoregulation may be caused by atherosclerotic changes, with or without vessel narrowing. A normal endothelium has more recently been described to be essential for the adjustments of the coronary artery diameter to the metabolic demand (6, 27). A number of vasodilator and vasoconstrictor factors released from the endothelial cells counteract to adjust the vessel diameter. In presence of endothelial damage there will be an inappropriate release of the vasodilating factors in relation to the vasoconstricting; it also comes from the circulating blood cells (3). Under most conditions, however, heart rate and rate of intraventricular pressure development are of major importance as triggering factors for the anginal attack.

Experience with β-blockers and calcium channel blockers

β-blockers have been used in the treatment of angina pectoris for more than 20 years. Somewhat later, the first calcium channel blocker, verapamil, was introduced. Most patients with angina pectoris have responded favorably to these medications (3, 23). Exercise capacity and the need for short-acting nitrates have been improved markedly in a very large number of placebo-controlled trials (7). The most important mechanism in explaining these results is the heart-rate reduction observed during physical and mental stress. The blunted heart-rate response in relation to a given exercise stress-test workload will allow a higher level of work before ischemic chest pain is induced (Fig. 1). The pressure development is also reduced, but this is of less importance in most cases. The heart-rate reduction at a given workload will reduce the coronary supply due to reduced metabolic demand. A lower heart rate will also prolong the diastolic perfusion period, which will favor coronary artery supply. The time for ventricular filling will also be longer, which will counteract the ischemia-induced stiffness of the myocardium during diastole (1).

Contraindications in the use of β-blockers and calcium channel blockers in the treatment of patients with angina pectoris are that they cause several adverse reactions. Symptoms of hypotension, low cardiac output or congestive heart failure may all be due to the reduction of heart rate *per se*. However, additional effects may be caused by a reduction of contractility from these drugs. There are also extracardiac adverse reactions to these treatments, e.g., on mental alertness, bronchial obstruction, and obstipation. A new class of drugs which would only affect heart rate will most likely be a valuable addition to the present therapy of angina pectoris.

Effects of β-blockers and calcium channel blockers on other ischemic events

β-blockers given intravenously to patients with unstable acute angina pectoris or with suspected acute myocardial infarction were found to cause several beneficial effects, as early as 15 years ago. There was reduction of ongoing severity of chest pain and of ST-segment elevation or depression (15, 28). These effects were more marked among patients with higher pretreatment heart rates. The addition of a β-blocker also caused a more marked fall in heart rate in these patients. Later, large

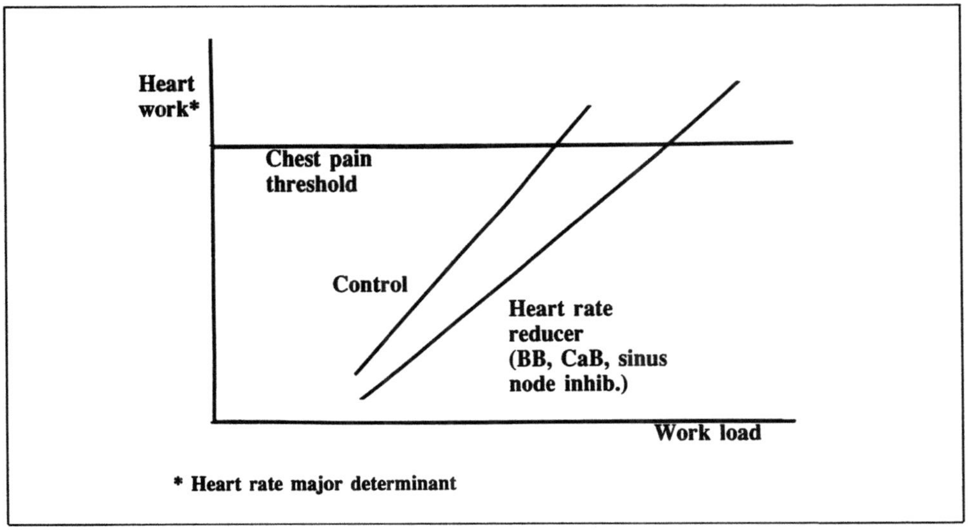

Fig. 1. Heart-rate reduction by β-blockers, calcium blockers or sinus node inhibitors will reduce heart work at a given workload, thus allowing an increased working capacity before the chest pain threshold is reached.

placebo-controlled trials have shown that some β-blockers also can limit and prevent infarct development. In the Göteborg Metoprolol Trial and the MIAMI Trial (2, 15, 22, 28), the favorable effects of metoprolol on chest pain, ST-segment changes, and on infarct development (enzymes and Q- and R-wave changes) were more marked in patients with higher initial heart rate and systolic blood pressure (Table 1). Pooled data of all published randomized trials on β-blockers after myocardial infarction have shown a 25 % reduction of reinfarctions later on (31). This effect was also related to entry heart rate (9).

Pooled data from 50 trials in about 50 000 patients have shown that β-blockers can reduce mortality early and late after myocardial infarction (12). It was also reported that the effect on mortality was more marked among patients with higher heart rate at entry (15; Fig. 2). Among these patients, heart rate was more reduced by the β-blocker therapy. It was proposed that the lowering of heart rate was correlated to the mortality reduction in the postinfarction trials (17; Fig. 3).

Calcium channel blockers have also been extensively studied in unstable angina pectoris and after myocardial infarction. There has been a total of 28 randomized trials with 19 000 patients. In a recent review (10), it was concluded that calcium channel blockers do not reduce the risk of initial or recurrent infarction or death when given to these patients. Furthermore, the authors of the review claimed that there is no conclusive evidence that calcium channel blockers can limit initial infarct development or reduce mortality or reinfarction in any particular subgroup of

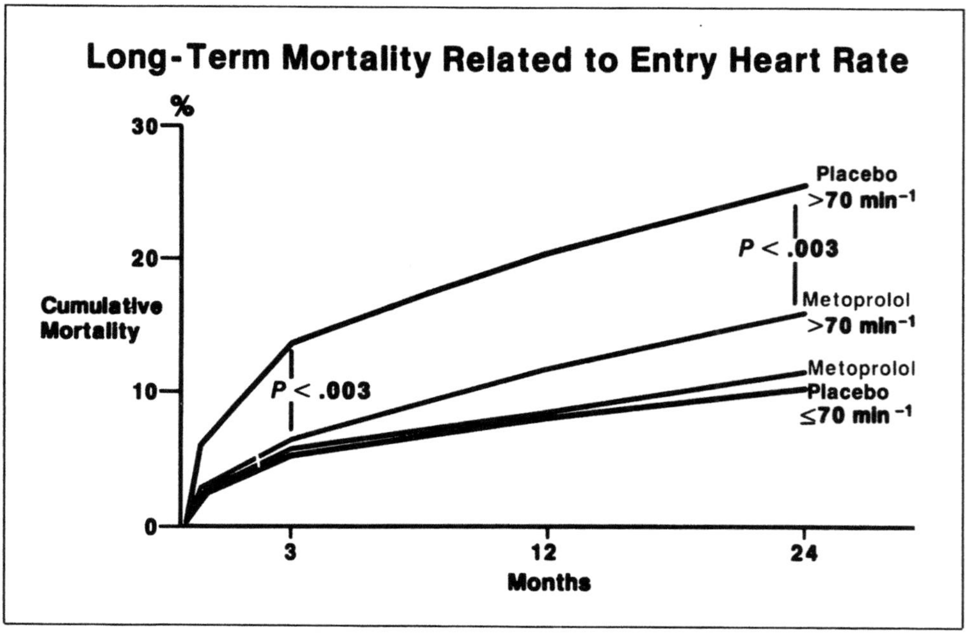

Fig. 2. Cumulative mortality in all patients during 2 years in the Göteborg Metoprolol Trial (12); blind medication (placebo and metoprolol) was given for 3 months and, thereafter, all patients were given the same treatment, most on open metoprolol. Mortality is significantly higher among patients who had a higher heart rate shortly after arrival in hospital before inclusion into the trial.

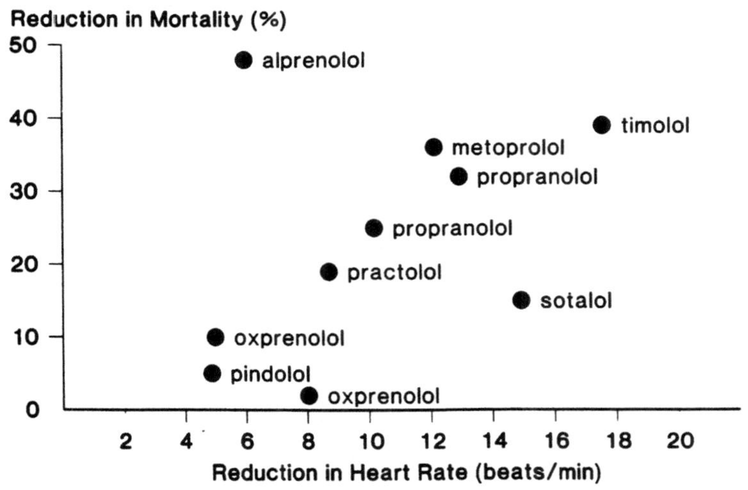

Fig. 3. Correlation between heart-rate reduction and mortality reduction in major studies comparing β-blockers and placebo after myocardial infarction (17).

patients (e.g., non-Q wave infarctions). The data on reinfarction were available from three trials of verapamil (3465 patients) and four trials of diltiazem (3117 patients), and there was a trend towards fewer reinfarctions in patients treated with verapamil and diltiazem. Nifedipin was studied in 12 trials (n = 7,325) with no trend of reinfarctions. Since this review, the second Danish Verapamil Infarction Trial was reported (25). Verapamil (n = 878) compared to placebo (n = 897) from 2 weeks postinfarction and continued for 18 months, significantly reduced first reinfarction ($p < 0.04$) and first cardiac event (death or reinfarction; $p < 0.03$). Mortality was not significantly reduced, although there was a favorable trend ($p = 0.11$). It can be concluded that the only calcium blocker presenting shown to have a favorable effect on infarct development or cardiovascular death is verapamil. Verapamil, in contrast to several other calcium blockers, has a property which reduces heart rate, similar to that seen with β-blockers.

Heart rate as a predictor in acute myocardial infarction

Elevated heart rate is a predictor of the risk of developing acute myocardial infarction and death. This is reported in several studies on primary and secondary prevention (5, 8, 14, 18, 26). The elevated heart rate has generally been considered to be a marker of depressed left-ventricular heart function and, especially, in studies of patients who suffered acute myocardial infarction. However several reports have reported that increased heart rate is an independent predictor of mortality (5, 8, 14, 18, 26). Heart rate *per se* has received little attention as a risk factor in the practical treatment of patients with acute myocardial infarction. In a number of trials on short- and long-term treatments with β-blockers in patients with acute myocardial infarction, mortality tended to be higher, with higher heart rate at entry to the trial (2, 9, 13, 15, 24). In one of the postinfarction trials, the Norwegian Timolol Multicenter Study (9), a logistic regression analysis was performed and showed that heart rate was a significant predictor of long-term mortality among patients treated with timolol, as well as with placebo, A pooling of randomized long-term placebo-controlled trials on β-blockers in postinfarction patients also showed that mortality after 1 to 2 years of myocardial infarction was higher among those with higher heart rate shortly after their infarction (31).

In one recent trial (14), a careful analysis was done to characterize, in a large population, the relationship between heart rate among patients with acute myocardial infarction and mortality. In this study of 1 807 patients of all ages with acute myocardial infarction admitted to hospital within 24 h of chest pain, the level of heart rate at hospital admission, maximal heart rate during the coronary care unit stay and at discharge were significantly related to in-hospital and post-discharge mortality. The trend for increased mortality with increasing heart rate appeared most pronounced in patients with absent to mild, or moderate heart failure. The total 1-year mortality for patients with admission heart rate ≥90 beats/min and absent to mild heart failure was 25 % compared to 10 % ($p < 0.001$) for patients with admission heart rate <90 beats/min. In this study, cumulative mortality from day 2 to 1 year was related to variables from the history and clinical course, using Cox regression analysis to identify independent predictors of one-year mortality. Admission heart rate was, among all known prognostic factors, fourth in rank according to its adjusted chi-square value ($p < 0.0004$), and was behind degree of heart failure, age, and maximal blood urea nitrogen.

In several studies on early β-blocker treatment in patients with suspected acute myocardial infarction, heart rate on arrival to hospital was not only a predictor of later mortality, but these patients also had more complications (11, 13, 15). Patients with higher heart rate tended to have more severe chest pain with a longer duration of pain, as well as a higher use of morphine analgesics. The patients with higher heart rate at entry also had signs of larger infarctions as estimated from enzymes and Q- and R-wave changes, and also more often developed a definite acute myocardial infarction compared to those with lower entry heart rates. Arrhythmias during hospital stay, including supraventricular and ventricular arrhythmias, were more frequently seen among patients with higher heart rates on arrival to hospital.

Conclusion

Reduction of heart rate is not a new concept in treating patients with angina pectoris. Most patients with angina pectoris experience pain during physical exercise or mental stress, which is known to cause an increase in heart rate and systolic blood pressure. Heart rate is a major determinant of cardiac oxygen consumption. The β-blockers and the calcium blocker verapamil have well known beneficial effects in patients with angina pectoris. One major mechanism of action is a reduction in heart rate caused by these agents. The introduction of a new type of medical therapy utilizing the sinus node inhibitors would therefore most likely be of great value. Combined treatments with various drugs might reduce heart rate further and prevent ischemic chest pain.

Heart rate has been reported to be a risk predictor for infarct development and death in primary as well as in secondary preventive studies. Prophylactic institution of β-blockers after onset of acute myocardial infarction and also in the primary prevention of patients with hypertension (28) have been found to reduce mortality and morbidity. In the secondary preventive studies the effects of morbidity and mortality by β-blockers were more marked in patients with higher heart rate at entry. Heart rate reduction might therefore be of importance for long-term prognosis.

β-blockers and calcium blockers are well established in the therapy of angina pectoris, and heartrate reduction in stress situations seems to be of great importance. In addition, β-blockers are recommended to be used for cardioprotection in patients who have suffered acute myocardial infarction, as well as in the primary prevention of patients with hypertension. Heartrate reduction may play an important role also for the cardioprotective effects of β-blockers. New bradycardic agents, such as the sinus node inhibitors, may be of value in the treatment of patients with various forms of ischemic heart disease both as mono therapy or combined with other antiischemic agents (16).

References

1. Barry WH, Brooker JZ, Alderman EL, Harrison DC (1974) Changes in diastolic stiffness and tone of the left ventricle during angina pectoris. Circulation 49: 255–263
2. Beta-blocker Heart Attack Trial Research Group (1982) A randomized trial of propranolol in patients with acute myocardial infarction. I. Mortality results. JAMA 247: 1707–1714
3. Chierchia S, Genosa S, Grazier JJ (1987) Beta-blockers for the treatment of angina pectoris, indications in relation to pathophysiological mechanisms. J Cardiovasc Pharmacol 10: 529–533
4. Collin P, Fox KM (1990) Pathophysiology of angina. Lancet i: 94–96
5. Coronary Drug Project Research Group (1974) Factors influencing long-term prognosis after recovery from myocardial infarction – three-year findings of the Coronary Drug project. J Chron Dist 27: 267–285
6. Davies PF, Olesen S-P, Clapham DE, Morrel EM, Schoen FJ (1988) Endothelial communication. State of the art lecture. Hypertension 11 (6) part 2: 563–572
7. Frishman WH (1986) Beta adrenergic blockade for the treatment of angina pectoris. In: Weiner D, Frishman WD (eds): Therapy of angina pectoris. New York, Marcel Dekker Inc
8. Gilpin E, Olshen R, Henning H, Ross J Jr (1983) Risk prediction after myocardial infarction, comparison of three multivariate methodologies. Cardiology 70: 73–84
9. Gundersen T, Gottum P, Pedersen T, Kjekshus KJ for the Norwegian Multicenter Study Group (1986) Effect of timolol on mortality and reinfarction after acute myocardial infarction: Prognostic importance of heart rate at rest. Am J Cardiol 58: 20–25
10. Held PH, Yusuf S, Furberg DC (1989) Calcium channel blockers in acute myocardial infarction and unstable angina: an overview. BMJ 299: 1187–1192
11. Herlitz J, Hjalmarson Å (1986) The role of beta-blockade in the limitation of infarct development. Br Heart J 7: 916–924
12. Hjalmarson Å (1991) Cardioprotection after myocardial infarction. Clin Cardiol. Accepted for publication
13. Hjalmarson Å for the MIAMI Trial Research Project (1985) MIAMI: Metoprolol in Acute Myocardial Infarction. Am J Cardiol 56: IG-57G
14. Hjalmarson Å, Gilpin EA, Kjekshus J, Schieman G, Nicod P, Henning H, Ross J Jr (1990) Influence of heart rate on mortality after acute myocardial infarction. Am J Cardiol 65: 547–553

15. Hjalmarson Å, Herlitz J (1984) The Göteborg Metoprolol Trial in acute myocardial infarction. Am J Cardiol 53: 1D–50D
16. Indolfi C, Guth BD, Miura T, Miyazaki S, Schulz R, Ross J Jr (1989) Mechanisms of improved ischemic regional dysfunction by bradycardia. Studies on UL-FS49 in swine. Circulation 80: 983–993
17. Kjekshus J (1987) Heart rate reduction – a mechanism of benefit? Eur Heart J 8 (suppl L): 115–122
18. Madsen EB, Gilpin E, Henning H, Ahnve S, LeWinter M, Ceretto W, Joswig W, Collins D, Pitt W, Ross J Jr (1984) Prediction of late mortality after myocardial infarction from variables measures at different times during hospitalization. Am J Cardiol 53: 47–54
19. Maseri A, Chierchia S, Kaski JC (1985) Mixed angina pectoris. Am J Cardiol 56: 30E–33E
20. Morris Jr JJ (1990) Mechanisms of ischemia in coronary artery disease: Spontaneou decrease in coronary blood supply. Am Heart J 120: 746–756
21. Nabel EG, Ganz P, Gordon JB, Alexander RW, Selwyn AP (1988) Dilation of normal and constriction of atherosclerotic coronary arteries caused by the cold pressor test. Circulation 77 (1): 43–52
22. Norwegian Multicenter Study Group (1981) Timolol-induced reduction in mortality and reinfarction in patients surviving acute myocardial infarction. N Engl J Med 304: 801–807
23. Packer M (1989) Drug therapy. Combined beta-adrenergic and calcium-entry blockade in angina pectoris. N Eng 1 J Med 320: 709–718
24. The Beta Blockeer Pooling Project (BBPP) (1988) Subgroup findings from randomized trials in postinfarction patients. Eur Heart J 9: 8–16
25. The Danish Study Group on Verapamil in Myocardial Infarction (1990) Effect of verapamil on mortality and major events after acute myocardial infarction (The Danish Verapamil Infarction Trial II - DAVIT II). Am J Cardiol 66: 779–785
26. Tibblin G, Eriksson C-G, Bjurö T, Georgescu D, Svärdsudd C (1975) Heart rate and heart rate variability a risk factor for the development of ischaemic heart disease (IHD) in the "men born in 1913 study" – a ten years follow-up. IRGS Medical Science: Cardiovascular System: Social and Occupational Medicine 3: 95.(abstr)
27. Vane JR, Änggård EE, Botting RM (1990) Regulatory functions of the vascular endothelium. N Engl J Med 323 (1): 27–36
28. Waagstein F, Hjalmarson Å (1875) Double-blind study of the effect of cardioselective beta-blockade on chest pain in acute myocardial infarction. Acta Med Scand 587: 201–208
29. Wikstrand J, Warnold I, Olsson G, Tuomilehto J, Elmfeldt D, Berglund G; on behalf of the Advisory Committee (1988) Primary prevention with metoprolol in patients with hypertension. Mortality results from the MAPHY Study. JAMA 259 (13) 1976–1982
30. Willerson JT, Golino P, Eidt J, Campbell WB, Buja LM (1989) Specific platelet mediators and unstable coronary artery lesions. Experimental evidence and potential clinical implications. Circulation 80: 198–205

Author's address:
Åke Hjalmarson, MD
Division of Cardiology,
Sahlgren's Hospital,
S-41345 Göteborg, Sweden

ULFS 49 CL, a prototype of a novel pharmacological concept

C. Lillie

Bender+Co Ges mbH, Research and Development, Vienna, Austria

Introduction

In patients with stable angina pectoris, ischemic attacks during exercise or other stress are caused by an imbalance between myocardial oxygen demand and oxygen supply. Current anti-ischemic drug therapy is aimed to extend exercise tolerance by an improvement of the O_2-demand/supply ratio. Antianginal drugs have been traditionally categorized as vasodilators mainly increasing O_2-supply (e.g., calcium-channel blockers, nitrates) and heart-rate-reducing drugs (e.g., β-adrenoceptor blockers), or combinations thereof (e.g., verapamil or diltiazem-like calcium-channel blockers). The conventional view of the mechanism of action of β-adrenoceptor blockers is relief of ischemia by a decrease of myocardial O_2-demand during exercise due to reductions of heart rate and contractility. However, the benefit of the negative inotropic effect of β-adrenoceptor blockers remains in dispute. The attenuation of exercise-induced tachycardia and the preservation of an adequate diastolic perfusion time was often suggested as the only therapeutic principle of β-adrenoceptor blockers.

In view of this controversy, the research department of Dr. Karl Thomae GmbH, Biberach, FRG, together with the pharmacological laboratory at the Ernst-Boehringer Institute in Vienna, Austria, in 1973, initiated a drug research program targeted towards compounds which selectively reduce heart rate without affecting cardiac contractility, conduction velocity and refractoriness, or arterial blood pressure. In fact, structural modification of the calcium-channel blocker verapamil led to a prototype with such a pharmacological profile, the benzolactame-derivative falipamil (AQ-A 39, Fig. 1). Due to its distinctive pharmacological pattern, the drug was termed a "specific bradycardic agent" (2, 13). Further optimization resulted in various active agents (25), the benzazepinone-derivative ULFS 49 CL (Fig. 1; rINN: zatebradine; 1,3,4,5-tetrahydro-7,8-dimethoxy-3-[3-[[2-(3,4-dimethoxyphenyl)ethyl]methylimino]propyl]-2H-3-benzazepin-2-on hydrochloride) became a new standard because of its increased potency, specificity, and prolonged duration of action (15, 17, 21).

Meanwhile, compounds of different chemical structures have been found to fit to the pharmacological classification of "specific bradycardic agents" (12, 16). The clonidine-derivative alinidine represented the first agent which showed this profile, not only in animals, but also in man; it also proved to be of benefit to patients with angina by reducing nitrate consumption and increasing maximum symptom-free

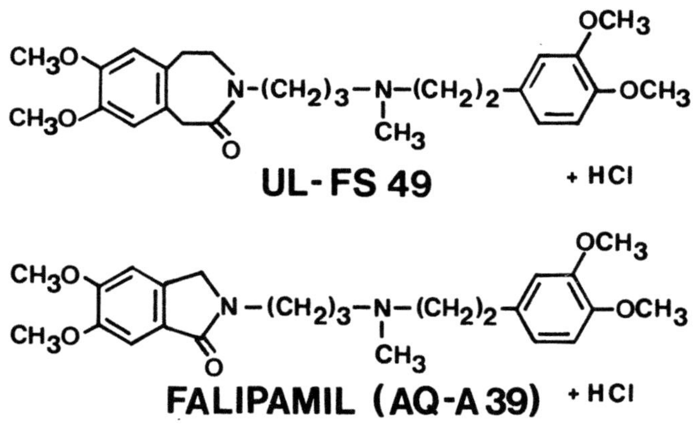

MW	log P	pK_a
493	0.66	8.73
465	0.43	8.58

Fig. 1. Chemical structures of ULFS 49 CL and falipamil. MW, molecular weight; log P, logarithm of the partition coefficient octanol/buffer, pH 7.4; pK_a, dissociation constant.

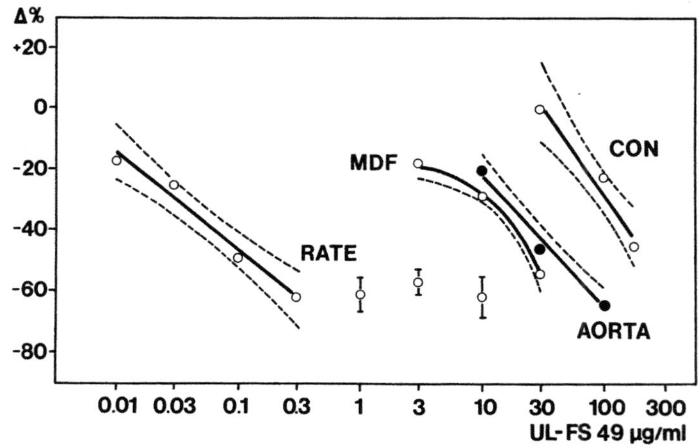

Fig. 2. Effects of ULFS 49 CL on spontaneous rate (RATE), maximal driving frequency (MDF) and contractility (CON) (electrical stimulation 2.5 Hz) in isolated guinea-pig atria, as well as on K^+-induced contracture in isolated aortic strips of rabbits (AORTA). Abscissa: concentration of ULFS 49 CL in the organ bath. Ordinate: drug-induced changes in percent of control values. Means of at least four experiments for each concentration. ○, atria, ●, aorta, Variability was estimated either by S.E. (vertical bars) or by 95 % confidence limits (dotted lines) of regression lines. (From Kobinger and Lillie (15).)

workload (10, 14). ULFS 49 CL, like alinidine, scientifically challenges not only physicians interested in the role of heart rate in ischemic heart disease, but also physiologists who use these drugs as tools for investigating the mechanism of the rhythmic discharges in the sinoatrial node. The following paragraphs summarize experimental features distinguishing agents like ULFS 49 CL from other cardioactive drugs, both with respect to the pharmacological profile and to the mode of action. Due to its slowing effect on spontaneous sinoatrial rate ULFS 49 CL sometimes is termed a “sinus node inhibitor”. However, ULFS 49 CL can clearly be differentiated from other drugs acting on the sinus node, such as calcium-channel blockers, antiarrhythmic and cholinergic agents.

Cardiovascular profile

Isolated Preparations

Figure 2 illustrates a set of results which initiated further development of ULFS 49 CL as a new standard for specific heart-rate reducing agents (15, 21). In isolated guinea-pig atria, ULFS 49 CL concentration-dependently decreased a) spontaneous sinus rate, as well as b) maximal driving frequency – as a test for refractory period and conduction velocity – and c) contractile force of electrically driven left atria. A vasorelaxant effect was found in isolated aortic strips of rabbits contracted in Tyrode’s solution with 42.7 mmol/L KCI and 1.8 mmol/L $CaCl_2$. The drug concentrations that reduced each parameter by 30 % (EC_{30}) were calculated. Table 1 gives the EC_{30} for the sinus rate reducing activity, the high ratios of the EC_{30}’s for the other three effects compared to the bradycardic EC_{30} express the high specificity of ULFS 49 CL for the effect on sinus rate.

Compared to other specific heart-rate-reducing agents tested before (alinidine, falipamil), ULFS 49 CL appeared as the most potent and also the most specific agent, as measured by the three ratios (Table 1). Calcium-channel blockers (verapamil, nifedipine, diltiazem) clearly differ from ULFS 49 CL because of their pronounced vasorelaxing activities (low ratios AORTA/RATE), antiarrhythmic drugs like mexiletine predominently reduce maximal driving frequency (low ratio

Table 1. The effects of drugs on spontaneous rate (RATE), contractility (CON) and maximal driving frequency (MDF) in isolated guinea-pig atria and on K^+-induced (43 mmol/L) contracture in isolated aortic strips of rabbits (AORTA). EC_{30} = concentration which decreased predrug value by 30 %, evaluated from concentration-response curves as shown in Fig. 2. The effects of single concentrations were determined after an equilibration period of 60 min. Left: EC_{30} for RATE. Right: ratios of the EC_{30} for the other three effects versus RATE. Carbachol: AORTA not tested. (Data from Kobinger and Lillie (16))

Substance	Decrease in atrial rate EC_{30} µg/ml	Ratio of EC_{30}		
		CON/RATE	MDF/RATE	AORTA/RATE
Alinidine	2.0	23	8.3	20
Falipamil	0.61	150	16	35
ULFS 49 CL	0.030	3600	380	500
Verapamil	0.069	0.88	3.1	0.41
Nifedipine	0.11	0.14	>7.3	0.036
Diltiazem	0.14	20	32	0.53
Mexiletine	21	0.60	0.098	2.3
Carbachol	0.029	0.22	MDF increased	–

MDF/RATE). In atria, cholinergic agents (carbachol) differ from ULFS 49 CL by a pronounced negative inotropic effect and an increase in maximal driving frequency. Furthermore, low concentrations of atropine (0.05 μg/ml) strongly block the rate-lowering effect of carbachol, without affecting the concentration-response curve of ULFS 49 CL (16, 17).

The selectivity of low doses of ULFS 49 CL for reduction of spontaneous sinoatrial rate without concomitant negative inotropic effects is the basis for the interaction of ULFS 49 CL with β-adrenergic agonists (Fig. 3): in isolated spontaneously beating guinea-pig atria the concentration-response curves for the positive chronotropic effect of isoprenaline were shifted down to lower frequency values along the ordinate, but not in parallel to the right along the abscissa, as would be expected from competitive antagonists, e.g., β-adrenoceptor blocking agents (22). These results indicate rather a functional antagonism, which explains the observation that ULFS 49 CL also antagonized the positive chronotropic effects of histamine and theophylline, while propranolol was ineffective (22). In contrast to β-adrenoceptor blockers, ULFS 49 CL did not antagonize the positive inotropic effect of isoprenaline (Fig. 3, bottom).

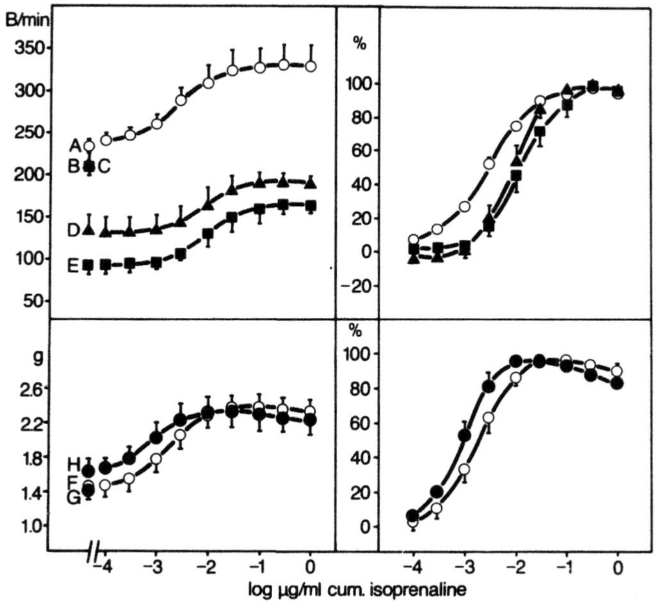

Fig. 3. Effects of cumulatively added isoprenaline in guinea-pig atria. Top: effect on rate of spontaneously beating atria. Control experiments (N = 9,○) or with ULFS 49 CL 0.03 μg/ml (n = 7,▲) or 0.1 μg/ml (n = 7,□). Bottom: effect on contractile force in electrically driven (1 Hz) left atria. Control experiments (n = 11, ○) or with ULFS 49 CL 1 μg/ml (n = 5,●). Abscissas: cumulative concentration of isoprenaline in the organ bath (log μg/ml). Ordinates: Left: atrial rate in beats/min (B/min) and isometric tension (g), respectively. A,B,C,F,G: values before addition of any drug; D,E,H: after ULFS 49 CL, before isoprenaline. Right: increases of rate and tension, respectivley, in percentage of the maximal effects reached by isoprenaline in each single experiment. Shown are mean values and S.E., whenever exceeding symbol size. (From Lillie and Kobinger (22).)

A comparison of ULFS 49 CL with propranolol in isolated guinea-pig atria prestimulated with isoprenaline (22) again revealed 1) the desired similarity to β-adrenoceptor blockers: the antagonism of the positive chronotropic effect of β-adrenergic stimulation, and 2) the presumably decisive therapeutic advantage over β-adrenoceptor blockers: no antagonism of the positive inotropic effect of β-adrenergic stimulation.

Intact animals

In intact animals, ULFS 49 CL reduced heart rate at doses which had little or no effect on other cardiovascular parameters such as arterial blood pressure, systemic vascular resistance, and left-ventricular contractility (+ dp/dt_{max}); stroke volume was rather increased (17, 20, 26). In anesthetized cats, prolongation of the diastolic period was the most prominent effect; ECG-parameters such as PQ- and QRS-intervals were not influenced. A prolongation of the QT-interval and the ventricular refractory period occured only to an extent which was expected and secondary to a pronounced heart-rate-reducing effect (15, 16). In these aspects, ULFS 49 CL contrasts with antiarrhythmics such as quinidine, which prolongs QRS-duration, and verapamil, which increases PQ-interval, or d-sotalol, which prolongs QT-interval and refractory period.

The potency of ULFS 49 CL with respect to heart-rate reduction differed in various species (17). In conscious dogs, one of the characteristic properties of ULFS 49 CL and related agents is a positive correlation between the control sinus rate and the extent of the rate-lowering effect (15). This "self-limiting" mechanism might explain why cardiac standstill or extreme bradycardia has not been reported.

In conscious and anesthetized dogs, the difference between ULFS 49 CL and β-adrenoceptor blockers, as demonstrated in isolated heart preparations, could be confirmed (20, 26). Of clinical interest is a comparison of the hemodynamic effects of ULFS 49 CL with those of propranolol in dogs, in doses with comparable reduction of exercise heart rate (Fig. 4; (20)). ULFS 49 CL (0.5 mg/kg i.v.) did not depress myocardial performance (rate of increase of left-ventricular pressure, cardiac output, left-ventricular stroke volume, and systolic wall thickening). Propranolol (1.0 mg/kg i.v.), in contrast to ULFS 49 CL, led to a marked reduction in positive dp/dt_{max}, stroke volume, and systolic wall thickening during exercise (and at rest; not shown). Additionally, propranolol decreased the exercise values of cardiac output to a far greater extent than ULFS 49 CL. There was no indication that ULFS 49 CL might impair the relaxation of the left ventricle: during exercise, in contrast to propranolol, ULFS 49 CL neither decreased stroke volume nor negative left-ventricular dp/dt_{max}.

Experimental myocardial ischemia

Decreases in signs of myocardial ischemia by pretreatment with specific heart-rate-reducing agents were already demonstrated in the first reports on alinidine and falipamil (13, 18); similar results were gained with ULFS 49 CL (16). In anesthetized cats with repeated acute occlusion (1 min) of a branch of the left coronary

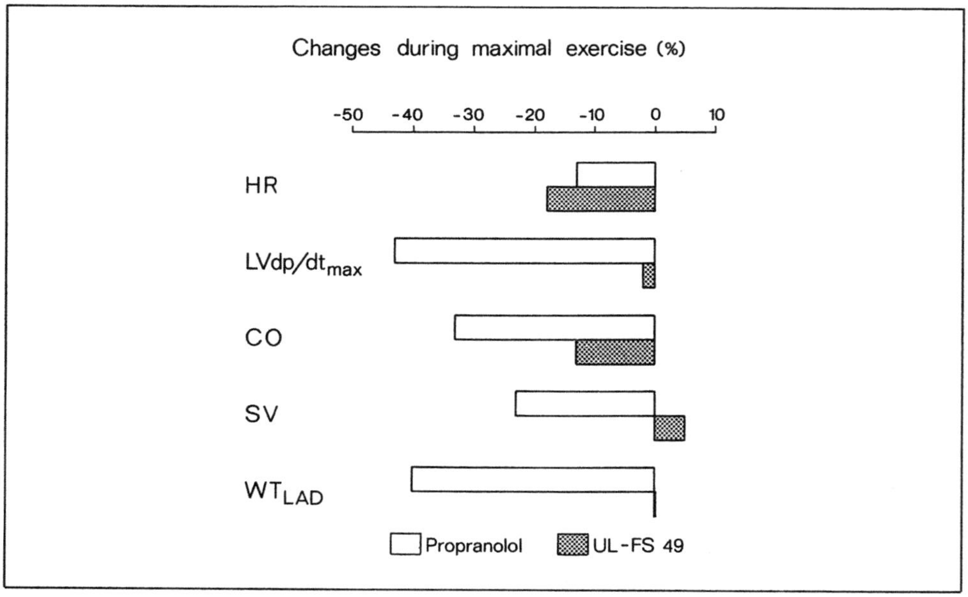

Fig. 4. Effects of ULFS 49 CL (0.5 mg/kg i.v.) and propranolol (1 mg/kg i.v.) on hemodynamic and functional parameters during treadmill exercise in dogs. Exercise at maximal work load: mean values of percentage changes after drug administration in comparison to the corresponding moment of control exercise (= 100%). Open columns: propranolol; hatched columns: ULFS 49 CL. Abbreviations: HR = heart rate, LV dp/dt_{max} = maximal rate of increase in left ventricular pressure, CO = cardiac output, SV = left-ventricular stroke volume, WT_{LAD} = left-ventricular systolic wall thickening. (By courtesy of G. Krumpl, Vienna; data from Krumpl et al. (20).)

artery, ULFS 49 CL, 0.5 mg/kg i.v., diminished ST-segment elevation in the epicardial electrogram.

Meanwhile, the effects of ULFS 49 CL on ischemic regional ventricular dysfunction have been studied extensively, both in anesthetized animals (3, 11) and in conscious dogs during exercise, with the aim of comparing ULFS 49 CL to β-adrenoceptor blockers (8, 19, 24). These studies are reviewed in detail in this volume (B.D. Guth, Chapter 3). In summary, the results suggest that heart-rate control during exercise is important for the prevention of ischemic regional myocardial dysfunction (27). Selective rate-lowering agents like ULFS 49 CL seem to have advantages over β-adrenoceptor blockers. The cardiodepressant effects of β-adrenoceptor blockers impair contractile function in non-ischemic regions during exercise and the reduction of arterial blood pressure impairs diastolic perfusion pressure. Both mechanisms counteract the beneficial effects of heart-rate control by β-adrenoceptor blockers.

Mode of action

The activity pattern of ULFS 49 CL in intact hearts (intact animals and isolated heart preparations) is based on a selective slowing effect on the spontaneous electrical depolarization in the pacemaker cells of the sinoatrial node, as

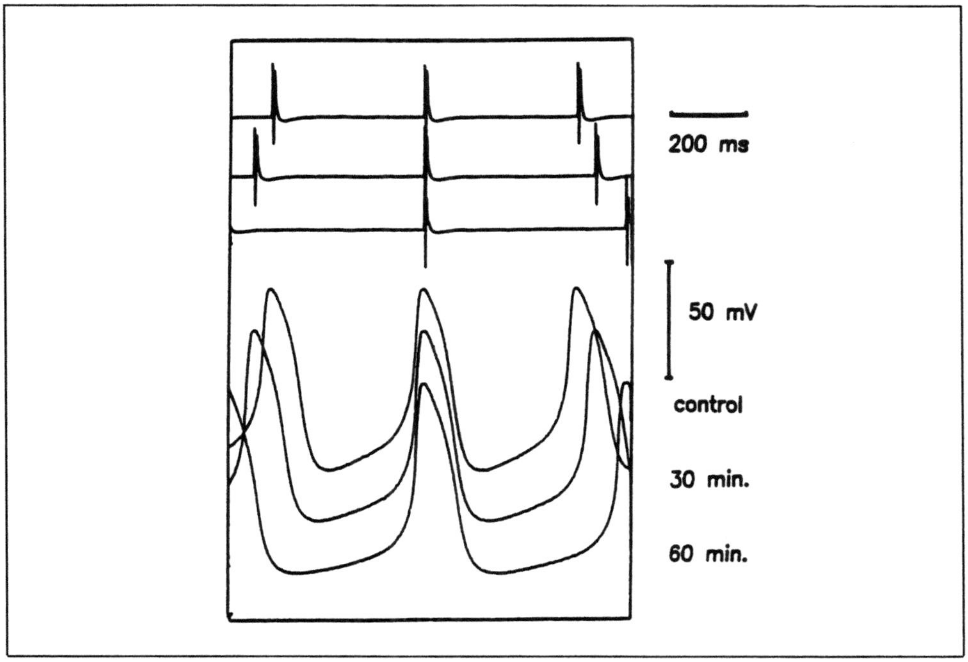

Fig. 5. Rabbit sinoatrial preparation, effect of ULFS 49 CL, 1.12 μmol/L. Top: electrograms of spontaneous discharges from the right atrium before (control) as well as 30 and 60 min after drug administration. Bottom: corresponding electrical activity of a dominant pacemaker fiber. For reproduction all curves were synchronized at the second discharge. (From Opt Hof and Bouman (23).)

determined by intracellular recordings (7, 31). Figure 5 shows this effect of ULFS 49 CL, 1.12 μmol/L, on transmembrane action potential (AP) configuration in electrograms of spontaneously beating rabbit sinoatrial preparations (23). Apparently, the rate of diastolic depolarization was reduced without concomitant effects on maximum diastolic potential, AP-amplitude, and AP-duration. A similar pattern was described in guinea-pig preparations, in which sinus-rate-lowering potency of ULFS 49 CL is higher than in rabbits: 0.04 μmol/L ULFS 49 CL significantly reduced the slope of slow diastolic depolarization in sinus node preparations, but did not change maximum diastolic potential, AP-amplitude, and AP-duration (7). An even higher concentration of ULFS 49 CL, 0.2 μmol/L, had no influence on resting potential, AP-amplitude, and maximum rate of rise of the AP in electrically driven guinea-pig left atria and papillary muscles (7).

The electrophysiological specificity of ULFS 49 CL towards diastolic depolarization rate is in agreement with the pharmacological profile as described in previous paragraphs: selective reduction of sinus rate without concomitant effects on cardiac contractility, conduction velocity, and refractoriness. In concentrations slowing spontaneous depolarization rate, other drugs have various other main effects on AP-configuration:

1) calcium-channel blockers decrease AP-amplitude in sinus node and depress the plateau-phase in both sinus node and contractile myocardium;

2) antiarrhythmic drugs, type quinidine or mexiletine, decrease maximum rate of rise of the AP in contractile myocardium and have various effects on AP-duration;
3) antiarrhythmic drugs, type d-sotalol, prolong AP-duration;
4) cholinergic agents shorten AP-duration and hyperpolarize the membane.

These electrophysiological patterns are the basis for the fact that sinus rate reduction is not the predominant effect of drugs of the classes 1)–4) (compare previous paragraphs).

There is no final answer yet to the question of which effect(s) of ULFS 49 CL on ionic membrane currents is underlying the decrease of diastolic depolarization rate in the intact sinoatrial node. Several different ionic currents contribute to spontaneous pacemaker depolarization (1, 9). Their relative role is still a matter of dispute, as experimental results strongly depend on the set-up. Effects of ULFS 49 CL on two ionic currents are discussed as being possibly responsible for the retarding effect on pacemaker depolarization:

1) A block of the L-type calcium inward current ($I_{Ca,L}$) by ULFS 49 CL observed in single sinoatrial node cells (6). This effect was frequency- and voltage-dependent and was much less pronounced in ventricular myocytes (6, 28). These observations are compatible with the lack of negative inotropy and of AV-conduction block in the intact heart. However, several pharmacological differences of ULFS 49 CL and related drugs to calcium-channel blockers are difficult to be reconciled with the hypothesis of a classical, verapamil-like blockade of $I_{Ca,L}$ as being the major effect of ULFS 49 CL (17). Such a hypothesis would also contrast with the following findings: in comparison to its chemical congener falipamil, ULFS 49 CL is about 20 times more potent in reducing sinoatrial rate (Table 1). Both drugs, however, show the same potency in blocking the classical $I_{Ca,L}$ (28).
2) In isolated cardiac Purkinje fibres, a selective inhibition of pacemaker current by ULFS 49 CL can clearly be attributed to a specific blockade of the hyperpolarization-activated Na/K-inward current "I_f" (or "I_h") 29, 30). The blockade is frequency- and voltage-dependent; ULFS 49 CL reaches a blocking site inside the I_f-channel from the cytoplasmic side of the membrane. This pattern conforms with the slow onset and disappearance of the drug action.

   In one set of experiments in sinoatrial node cells of rabbits, ULFS 49 CL conclusively blocked I_f, only in a rather high concentration; in guinea-pig cells, with one concentration of ULFS 49 CL no effect could be demonstrated (6). However, interpretation of these results is complicated by general difficulties in characterizing I_f in single sinoatrioal node cells, e.g., spontaneous current run-down (5, 6). The exact contribution of I_f to sinus pacemaking is still controversial, but recent results strongly indicate a modulatory role of I_f in the control of sinus pacemaker rate (4).

Due to its unique pharmacological properties, ULFS 49 CL in the future may serve as a tool for physiologists to elucidate the importance of various ionic currents for the maintenance of spontanous pacemaking in the human heart.

Conclusions

Data have been reviewed which suggest that ULFS 49 CL is a prototype of a novel class of drugs which have been termed "specific bradycardic agents" or "sinus node inhibitors". The predominant cardiovascular effect of these drugs is a slowing of the sinoatrial rate within physiological limits. The pharmacological profile of ULFS 49 CL clearly differs from that of other classes of drugs slowing sinus rate, such as calcium-channel blockers, antiarrhythmic and cholinergic agents. Such a difference was also established in electrophysiological experiments, where retardation of the diastolic depolarization rate in pacemaker cells was the main effect on cardiac action potentials. The specific mechanism of action of ULFS 49 CL on the level of ionic membrane currents needs further elucidation, the drug will provide new insight into the physiology of rhythmic discharges in pacemaker cells.

For the treatment of angina pectoris, ULFS 49 CL sems to have clear-cut advantages over other drugs following the concept of heart-rate reduction, such as β-adrenoceptor blockers. In doses with comparable reduction of a tachycardia induced by β-adrenergic stimulation, ULFS 49 CL does not antagonize the positive inotropic effect of this stimulation. ULFS 49 CL may serve as a tool for clinicians to explore the beneficial effect of selective sinus rate reduction in a variety of states with increased heart rates.

References

1. Brown HF (1982) Electrophysiology of the sinoatrial node. Physiol Rev 62: 505–530
2. Dämmgen J, Kadatz R, Diederen W (1981) Cardiovascular actions of 5,6-dimethoxy-2-[3[[α-(3,4-dimethoxy)-phenylethyl]-methylamino]propyl]phtalimidine (AQ-A 39), a specific bradycardic agent. Arzneim Forsch 31: 666–670
3. Dämmgen JW, Lamping KA, Gross GJ (1985) Actions of two new bradycardic agents, AQ-AH 208 and ULFS 49 CL, on ischemic myocardial perfusion and function. J Cardiovasc Pharmacol 7: 71–79
4. Denyer JC, Brown HF (1990) Pacemaking in rabbit isolated sino-atrial node cells during Cs^+ block of the hyperpolarization-activated current i_f. J Physiol (London) 429: 401–409
5. Di Francesco D, Ferroni A, Mazzanti M, Tromba C (1986) Properties of the hyperpolarizing-activated current (i_f) in cells isolated from the rabbit sino-atrial node. J Physiol (London) 377: 61–88
6. Doerr Th, Trautwein W (1990) On the mechanism of the "specific bradycardic action" of the verapamil derivative ULFS 49 CL. Naunyn Schmiedeberg's Arch Pharmacol 341: 331–340
7. Gruber R, Lumper G, Zilberszac A, Heistracher P (1983) Effects of 1,3,4,5-tetrahydro-7,8-dimethoxy-3-[3-[[2-(3,4-dimethoxyphenyl)ethyl]methylimino]propyl]-2H-3-benzazepin-2-on hydrochloride (ULFS 49 CL) on the action potential of the guinea-pig heart. Naunyn Schmiedeberg's Arch Pharmacol 324: R 32
8. Guth BD, Heusch G, Seitelberger R, Ross J Jr (1987) Elimination of exercise-induced myocardial dysfunction by a bradycardic agent in dogs with coronary artery stenosis. Circulation 75: 661–669
9. Hagiwara N, Irisaawa H, Kameyama M (1988) Contribution of two types of calcium currents to the pacemaker potentials of rabbit sino-atrial node cells. J Physiol (London) 395: 233–253
10. Harron DWG, Shanks RG (1985) Pharmacology, clinical pharmacology and potential therapeutic uses of the specific bradycardiac agent alinidine. Eur Heart J 6: 722–729
11. Indolfi C, Guth BD, Miura T, Miyazaki S, Schulz R, Ross J Jr (1989). Mechanisms of improved ischemic regional dysfunction by bradycardia. Studies on ULFS 49 CL in swine. Circulation 80: 983–993

12. Kobinger W (1989) Specific bradycardic agents. In: Vaughan Williams EM, Campbell TJ (eds) Handbook of experimental pharmacology, Vol. 89. Springer-Verlag, Berlin Heidelberg, pp 423–452
13. Kobinger W, Lillie C (1981) AQ-A 39 (5,6-dimethoxy-2[3[[α-(3,4-dimethoxy)phenylethyl]methylamino]propyl]phtalimidine), a specific bradycadic agent with direct action on the heart. Eur J Pharmacol 72: 153–164
14. Kobinger W, Lillie C (1984) Alinidine. In: Scriabine A (ed) New drugs annual: Cardiovascular drugs, vol 2. Raven Press, New York, pp 193–210
15. Kobinger W, Lillie C (1984) Cardiovascular characterization of ULFS 49 CL, 1,3,4,5-tetrahydro-7,8-dimethoxy-3-[3-[[2-(3,4-dimethoxyphenyl)ethyl]methylimino]propyl]-2H-3-benzazepin-2-on hydrochloride, a new "specific bradycardic agent". Eur J Pharmacol 104: 9–18
16. Kobinger W, Lillie C (1987) Specific bradycardic agents – a novel pharmacological class? Eur Heart J 8 (Suppl. L): 7–15
17. Kobinger W, Lillie C (1988) Falipamil (AQ-A 39) and ULFS 49 CL. Cardiovascular Drug Reviews 6: 35–53
18. Kobinger W, Lillie C, Pichler L (1979) Cardiovascular actions of N-allyl-clonidine (ST 567), a substance with specific bradycardic action. Eur J Pharmacol 58: 141–150
19. Krumpl G, Schneider W, Raberger G (1986) Can exercise-induced regional contractile dysfunction be prevented by selective bradycardic agents? Naunyn Schmiedeberg's Arch Pharmacol 334: 540–543
20. Krumpl G, Winkler M, Schneider W, Raberger G (1988) Comparison of the haemodynamic effects of the selective bradycardic agent ULFS 49 CL, with those of propranolol during treadmill exercise in dogs. Br J Pharmacol 94: 55–64
21. Lillie C, Kobinger W (1983) Cardiovascular actions of ULFS 49 CL, 1,3,4,5-tetrahydro-7,8-dimethoxy-3-[3-[[2-(3,4-dimethoxyphenyl)ethyl]methylimino]propyl]-2H-3-benzazepin-2-on hydrochloride, a new "specific bradycardic agent". Naunyn Schmiedeberg's Arch Pharamcol 324: R 33
22. Lillie C, Kobinger W (1986) Investigations into the bradycardic effects of ULFS 49 CL (1,3,4,5-tetrahydro-7,8-dimethoxy-3-[3-[[2-(3,4-dimethoxyhenyl)ethyl]methylimino]propyl]-2H-3-benzazepin-2-on hydrochloride) in isolated guinea pig atria. J Cardiovasc Pharmacol 8: 791–797
23. Opt Hof T, Bouman LN (1988) personal communication. In: Kobinger W, Lillie C. Falipamil (AQ-A 39) and ULFS 49 CL. Cardiovascular Drug Reviews 6: 35–53
24. Raberger G, Krumpl G, Schneider W (1987) Effects of the bradycardic agent ULFS 49 CL on exercise-induced regional contractile dysfunction in dogs. Int J Cardiol 14: 343–354
25. Reiffen M, Eberlein, W, Müller P, Psiorz M, Noll K, Heider J, Lillie C, Kobinger W, Luger P (1990) Specific bradycardic agents. 1. Chemistry, pharmacology, and structure-activity relationships of substituted benzazepinones, a new class of compounds exerting antiischemic properties. J Med Chem 33: 1496–1504
26. Riley DC, Gross GJ, Kampine KP, Warltier DC (1987) Specific bradycardic agents, a new therapeutic modality for anaesthesiology: hemodynamic effects of ULFS 49 CL and propranolol in conscious and isoflurane-anesthetized dogs. Anaesthesiology 67: 707–716
27. Ross J Jr (1989) Mechanisms of regional ischemia and antianginal drug action during exercise. Prog Cardiov Dis 31: 455–466
28. Tytgat J, Van Bogaert PP, Vereecke J, Carmeliet E (1990) Sensitivity of ventricular L-type Ca Channels to the bradycardic agents AQ-A 39, ULFS 49 CL and DK-AH 3. In: Vereeke J, Van Bogaert PP, Verdonck F (eds) Ionic currents and Ischemia. Leuven University Press, pp 276–278
29. Van Bogaert PP, Goethals M (1987) Pharmacological influence of specific bradycardic agents on the pacemaker current of sheep cardiac Purkinje fibres. A comparison between three different molecules. Eur Heart J 8 (Suppl. L): 35–42
30. Van Bogaert PP, Goethals M, Simoens C (1990) Use- and frequency-dependent blockade by ULFS 49 CL of the i_f pacemaker current in sheep cardiac Purkinje fibres. Eur. J Pharmacol 187: 241–256

31. Van Ginneken ACG, Bouman LN, Jongsma HJ, Duivenvoorden JJ, Opt Hof T, Giles WR (1987) Alinidine as a model of the mode of action of specific bradycardic agents on SA node activity. Eur Heart J 8 (Suppl. L): 25–33

Author's address:
Christian Lillie,
Bender+Co Ges mbH,
A-1121 Vienna, Austria

Sinus node inhibitors for reducing exercise-induced myocardial ischemia: Evidence from experimental animal studies

Brian D. Guth

Abteilung für Pathophysiologie, Universitätsklinikum Essen, FRG

Introduction

The physician is faced with the dilemma of how best to protect the myocardium subjected to effort-induced ischemia. The ultimate therapeutic solution is the elimination of the stenotic lesion. However, prior to vessel dilation or surgery (or in patients in which such procedures may not be advisable), treatment to minimize ischemic damage to the post-stenotic myocardium is indicated. The reduction of heart rate (or prevention of tachycardia) is an attractive therapeutic approach in the treatment of effort angina pectoris since it has a dual beneficial effect on the potentially ischemic post-stenotic myocardium. On the one hand, reduction of the number of contractions per minute of the heart reduces its work and, consequently, oxygen demand. At the same time, heart rate reduction acts to enhance myocardial blood flow and to improve its distribution within the ischemic myocardium by prolonging the diastolic interval and reducing coronary "steal". Thus, the inequality between an enhanced metabolic demand and a reduced nutritive supply is lessened from both sides of the supply-demand equation.

The purpose of this chapter is to review some of the pathophysiological aspects of effort-induced regional myocardial ischemia as determined through experimental animal studies. This will focus primarily on the role of tachycardia in the genesis and aggravation of regional myocardial ischemia. The importance of heartrate reduction in mediating the beneficial effect of β-adrenoceptor blockade in the setting of a fixed, single-vessel coronary stenosis will be assessed. Finally, experimental evidence supporting a role for sinus node inhibitors in treating effort-induced angina pectoris is reviewed.

Pathophysiological basis of effort-induced angina

Dynamic exercise necessitates an increase in total body oxygen consumption achieved through both an increased cardiac output and enhanced oxygen extraction

Dr. Guth is the recipient of a Research Fellowship from the Alexander von Humboldt-Stiftung, Bonn, FRG. Studies were supported in part by the National Institutes of Health Research Grant HL-17682, Ischemic Heart Disease Specialized Center of Research (SCOR) awarded by the National Heart, Lung and Blood Institute, Bethesda, MD.

in the working musculature. Increased cardiac output is a result of both tachycardia and increased stroke volume, made possible by activation of the sympathetic nervous system and an enhanced venous return. With this enhanced cardiac performance, myocardial oxygen demand can be increased over five-fold. The heart increases its oxygen consumption primarily through increases in oxygen delivery (increased blood flow), since the oxygen extraction in the heart is relatively high even at rest. Thus, a metabolically-induced reduction in coronary vascular resistance is responsible for increased blood flow and oxygen delivery to the working heart. The consequences of a flow-limiting coronary lesion on a large conduit artery in this setting, where blood flow would normally be greatly elevated, are dramatic. The effects on regional myocardial blood flow, its transmural distribution and regional contractile function will be considered next.

Regional myocardial blood flow and its distribution

A coronary arterial lesion can impose a pathological resistance on blood flow through the vessel, resulting in a decrease in post-stenotic coronary pressure. Blood flow to the myocardium can be maintained, despite such a drop in coronary perfusion pressure, in a perfusion bed capable of autoregulation; an autoregulating circulation will reduce its resistance to maintain flow despite the reduced perfusion pressure. In the resting conscious dog, autoregulation is effective down to perfusion pressures of approximately 40–50 mmHg [8]. Since coronary perfusion pressures are usually 80–120 mmHg (essentially proximal aortic pressure), this range of perfusion pressures over which the coronary vasculature can further vasodilate constitutes a vascular reserve and is termed its “autoregulatory reserve”. During exercise, however, the myocardium is already relatively vasodilated in order to provide the increased flow required by the increased cardiac work. This limits the ability of the coronary circulation to accommodate an abnormally low perfusion pressure distal to a coronary stenosis. When autoregulatory reserve becomes exhausted, blood flow to the tissue becomes directly dependent upon perfusion pressure. Thus, further decreases in coronary perfusion pressure produce ischemia, with the deeper, subendocardial layers most susceptible.

Blood flow to the left ventricle is nearly homogeneous across the wall under normal conditions. The ratio of subendocardial to subepicardial blood flow (“endo/epi ratio”) provides an index of this transmural distribution and normally varies from slightly less than 1.0 (anterior left ventricular wall of pigs [15, 22, 32, 40]) to somewhat greater than 1.0 (lateral left ventricular wall of dogs [1, 5, 7, 13]). The transmural homogeneity of blood flow is also maintained during severe dynamic exercise [2, 31]. However, tachycardia during exercise presents a mechanical problem for the perfusion of the inner ventricular wall, since cardiac contraction increases intramyocardial pressures, collapsing intramural vessels and, thereby, preventing blood flow during ventricular systole [9, 36]. Due to the gradient of intramyocardial pressure increasing from epicardium to endocardium [41], perfusion of the inner left ventricular wall is affected most. Perfusion of the inner layers of the left ventricular wall occurs almost entirely during ventricular diastole. Therefore, tachycardia and the resultant shortening of the diastolic interval impinges far greater upon subendocardial perfusion than on subepicardial perfusion [2, 5, 30, 31]. This has been demonstrated experimentally since heart rate and blood flow to the innermost left ventricular wall are inversely related in a non-autoregulating perfusion bed [3, 31]. With increasing tachycardia in a flow-limited perfusion bed, the normally homogeneous transmural blood flow is markedly altered such that the endo/epi ratio becomes greatly reduced [1, 5, 33, 34, 38]. In exercising dogs in which an acute stenosis of the circumflex coronary artery is imposed, a similar transmural redistribution of blood flow is observed, with the greatest reductions always occurring in the subendocardial region [13, 14].

Redistribution of blood flow during exercise (resulting in subendocardial ischemia) can also occur even when total coronary blood flow is not reduced. In dogs chronically instrumented with an ameroid constrictive device on the left circumflex coronary artery, a slowly progressing "fixed" coronary stenosis is created [15]. This is a useful experimental model for single-vessel coronary artery disease and has the advantage that the severity of the stenotic lesion is constant; the model is shown schematically in Fig. 1. In these dogs, studies can be performed at a time when the severity of the coronary stenosis does not affect perfusion of the wall during resting conditions, but it does limit exercise-induced hyperemia [20, 21]. Whereas total blood flow to the post-stenotic region remains constant (or may even increase slightly) during treadmill exercise in these dogs, subendocardial blood flow decreases substantially (Fig. 2). The loss of blood flow to the subendocardium is not only due to the mechanical disadvantage of perfusing the inner left ventricular wall because of the tachycardia, as discussed above, but also due to a transmural "steal"

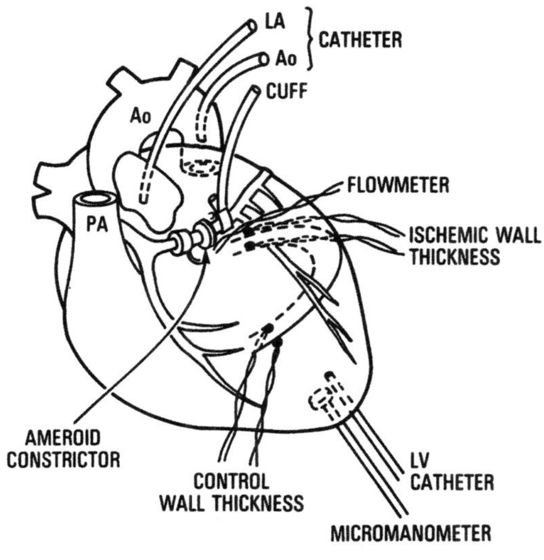

Fig. 1. Schematic diagram of the experimental model used in these studies. Dogs were chronically instrumented with wall-thickness gauges in the post-stenotic posterolateral wall and in the non-ischemic anterior wall of the left ventricle. Left ventricular pressure and its first derivative were measured using a high-fidelity pressure transducer in the left-ventricular chamber, calibrated by a fluid-filled catheter. The proximal left circumflex coronary artery was isolated and instrumented with a Doppler flow probe, an ameroid constrictor, and a pneumatic occlusive cuff. Catheters were placed in the descending thoracic aorta and left atrium for measuring blood flow by use of radiolabelled microspheres.

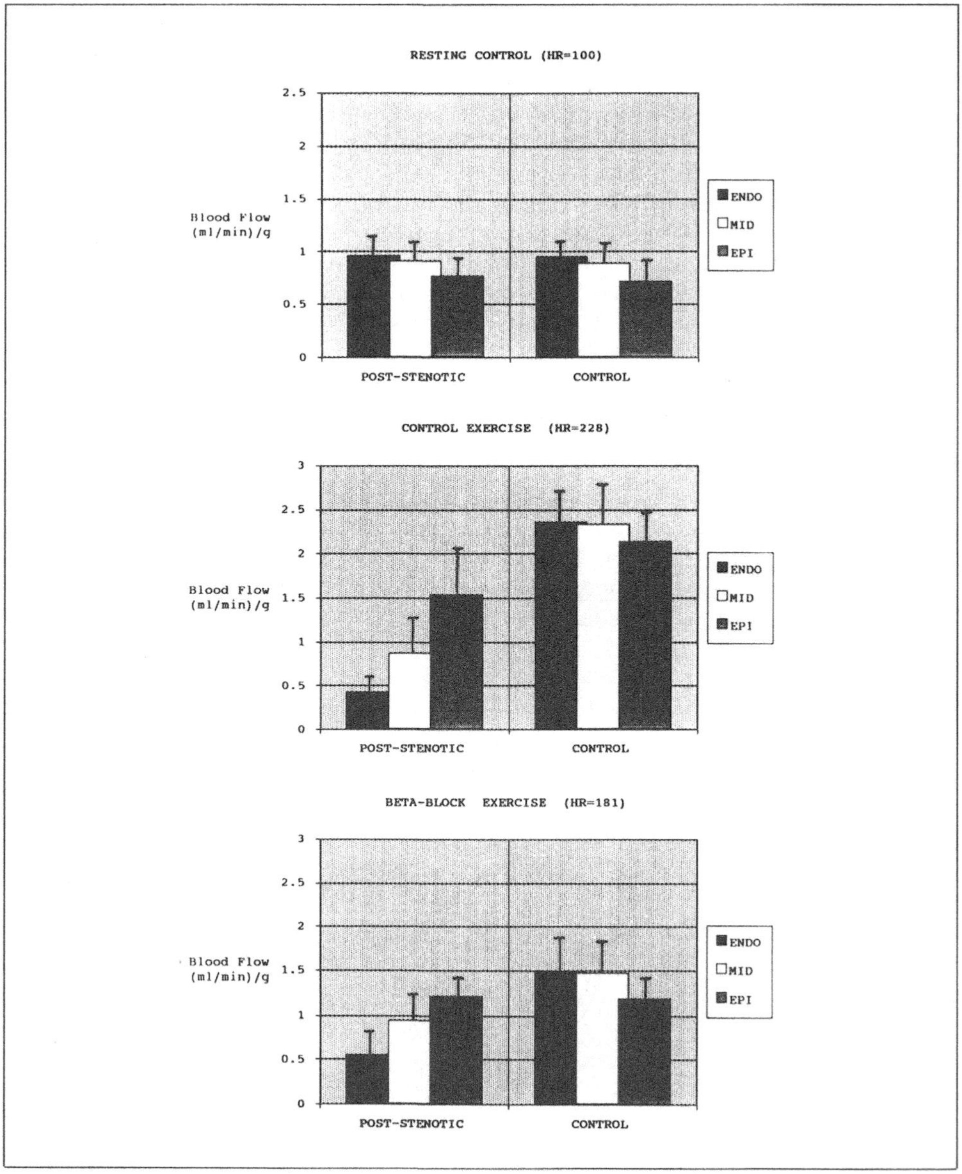

Fig. 2. Transmural distribution of regional myocardial blood flow in the ischemic, post-stenotic posterior wall (left panel) and control anterior wall (right panel) under resting conditions (upper middle), during control exercise before β-blockade (middle), and during exercise after β-blockade (bottom). For each condition, blood flow to the subendocardium (ENDO), midmyocardium (MID), and subepicardium (EPI) is given. Under resting conditions there is a homogeneous distribution of blood flow across both the anterior control wall and post-stenotic wall. During control exercise, blood flow to all transmural layers of the control wall increases, whereas there is a marked transmural redistribution in the post-stenotic wall. After β-blockade the ENDO blood flow in the post-stenotic region is increased, but blood flow to the outer wall and to the control wall is substantially decreased. Mean ± SD, N=9.

of blood flow from the subendocardium to the outer left ventricular wall [11, 13]. Transmural *steal* occurs because metabolic vasodilation of the coronary resistance vessels in the outer layers of the myocardium during exercise produces a decrease in post-stenotic perfusion pressure. This further fall in perfusion pressure causes an additional decrease in blood flow to the inner wall because its perfusion is pressure-dependent since its autoregulatory capacity has been exhausted by the already low post-stenotic coronary pressure. In arteries perfusing both left ventricular and right ventricular tissue, coronary *steal* may also occur from the left to the right ventricular portion of the bed to exacerbate ischemia in the left ventricular subendocardium [22]. Such *interventricular steal,* recently described in swine, is likely caused by metabolic vasodilation within the right ventricular myocardium persisting at perfusion pressures so low that the left ventricular subendocardial vasculature is pressure-dependent [29]. Thus, the myocardial bloodflow defect occurring during exercise-induced ischemia is not only based on the inability of flow to increase in order to match the increased metabolic demands, but also due to *steal* mechanisms which are active in actually reducing blood flow to the inner leftventricular wall.

Regional myocardial function during effort-induced angina

The profound effects of such bloodflow impairment on the contractile function of the post-stenotic myocardium have been thoroughly described in experimental studies [12, 13, 43]. Regional contractile performance of the heart has been measured in chronically-instrumented dogs using an ultrasonic technique [13, 43]. Increases in leftventricular wallthickening during ventricular systole have been shown to be a useful indicator of the contractile state of the myocardium [39], and are analogous to measurements of regional wallthickening made in man using echocardiography. In resting dogs subjected to an acute coronary stenosis, there is a nearly linear relationship between the decrease in blood flow and the decrease in regional contractile function [12, 43]. A linear relationship between decreased blood flow and decreased function has also been observed in exercising dogs with an acute coronary artery stenosis [13]. However, the relation is shifted during exercise such that a given level of blood flow per minute is associated with less regional function. However, if one instead considers the amount of blood flow *per heart beat* (as opposed to blood flow per minute), there appears to be a close relationship to the contractile function of the ischemic region which is similar at rest and during exercise [13]. Such a relationship existing both at rest and during exercise is perhaps surprising, since other determinants of myocardial oxygen consumption, including afterload and preload, are not considered. Nevertheless, for predicting the regional contractile function during acute myocardial ischemia, the ratio between blood flow (oxygen supply) and heart rate (demand) would appear to be adequate [25].

Exercise-induced ischemia as a supply-demand imbalance

Ischemia has been described as a condition where the oxygen demand is not adequately matched by oxygen supply, i.e., there is a supply-demand imbalance

[37]. In the initial stages of exercise-induced ischemia this is undoubtedly the case. With the onset of treadmill exercise, dogs with chronic single-vessel coronary stenosis respond with an immediate increase in heart rate and regional contractile function, even in the post-stenotic region. Both increased heart rate and increased contractile performance are indicative of an increase in myocardial oxygen demand. However, due to the presence of the coronary stenosis, blood flow cannot increase as it normally would, leading to an initial supply-demand imbalance. The regional contractile function of the hypoperfused myocardium rapidly deteriorates and the severity of the subsequent steady-state ischemic dysfunction is directly related to the severity of the hypoperfusion [14]. The disparity of the initial supply-demand imbalance, however, has been lessened by the loss of contractile performance in the ischemic, post-stenotic region. Oxygen consumption, therefore, becomes limited by oxygen delivery. This has been termed a perfusion-contraction "matching" during acute, steady-state regional myocardial ischemia [37]. It is not reasonable to assume that myocardial supply and demand are once again adequately matched in this setting since ischemia-induced contractile dysfunction is indicative of pathological metabolic derangements in the ischemic myocardium that will eventually result in myocardial cell death. It can, however, be argued that the loss of regional contractile performance does serve to minimize the discrepancy between oxygen supply and demand, thereby allowing the myocardium to withstand longer periods of ischemia without permanent damage than would be possible if contractile function were preserved during ischemia [37].

The importance of these conceptual considerations to the clinician lies with the observation that the ratio between blood flow to the myocardium and heart rate is a close correlate to the severity of ischemia [25]. This ratio can be improved either

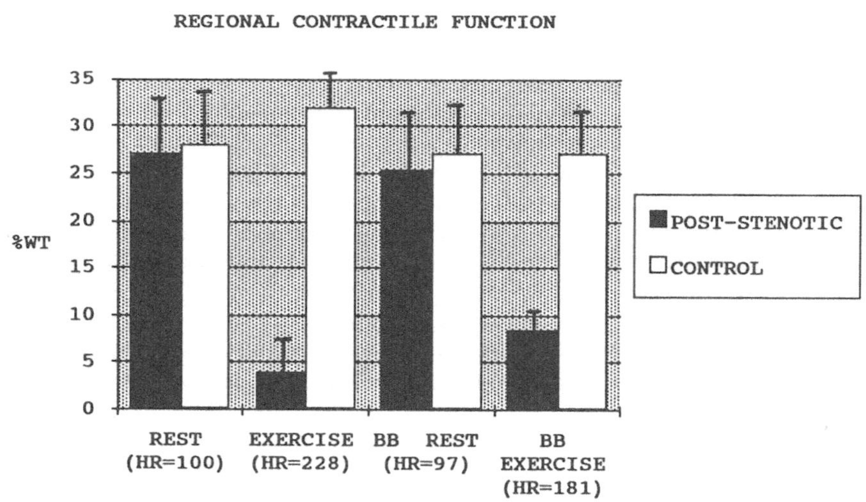

Fig. 3. Summary of regional wallthickening data during exercise before and after β-blockade. During the control exercise, wallthickening in the post-stenotic region was substantially reduced, whereas it increased in the control wall. In the run following β-blockade, wallthickening in the post-stenotic region was slightly improved, but control wall function was also depressed in comparison to the control run.

through increases in blood flow or a reduction in heart rate. As mentioned in the Introduction, treatment of ischemic heart disease ultimately requires the removal of the stenotic lesion so that blood flow is unhindered. However, prior to such intervention, reduction of heart rate or prevention of tachycardia would appear to be of major benefit to the patient. The importance of heartrate reduction to the beneficial effects of β-adrenoceptor blockade on exercise-induced ischemia will be evaluated next.

β-Adrenoceptor blockade for reducing exercise-induced ischemia

The blockade of β-adrenoceptors has become a frontline treatment for effort angina pectoris [10, 24, 44]. β-Blockade results in both negative inotropic and chronotropic effects and has been shown to improve blood flow and function in dogs distal to an acute coronary artery stenosis [6, 7, 18, 42]. β-Blockade markedly alters the hemodynamic response to treadmill exercise in dogs by reducing the heartrate response and by inhibiting the normal increase in inotropic state [3]. Overall, such an effect has been shown to be clearly beneficial during effort-induced ischemia in experimental studies designed to model human, single-vessel, coronary artery disease [27, 28].

In dogs with single-vessel, chronic coronary artery stenosis produced with an ameroid constrictor, two identical treadmill runs (same treadmill speed, inclination and duration) performed 3 h apart have been shown to be completely reproducible in terms of the hemodynamic response, the amount of ischemia induced, and the resultant contractile dysfunction [26]. This indicates that the severity of stenosis and the development of coronary collateral vessels does not change appreciably over this time period. The model allows for the evaluation of pharmacologic agents by treating the animals prior to the second exercise bout. In one such study designed to test the β-blocker atenolol, submaximal treadmill exercise producing a heart rate of 218 bpm was associated with subendocardial ischemia in the post-stenotic region (Fig. 2) and severe regional contractile dysfunction (Fig. 3) [28]. Ischemia was most predominant in the subendocardial region with an *increase* in blood flow to the outer layers of the post-stenotic region, thereby demonstrating transmural *steal* (Fig. 2). Before the second, experimental run, dogs were β-blocked (atenolol, 100 mg p.o.). In the run following β-blockade, heart rate during exercise was reduced to 166 bpm and contractile function in a non-ischemic region was depressed, indicative of the negative chronotropic and inotropic effects of the drug. However, blood flow to the ischemic subendocardium was increased (Fig. 2) as was post-stenotic regional contractile function (Fig. 3). Thus, β-blockade was shown to be effective in the reduction of exercise-induced ischemia. In a subsequent study, combined treatment of atenolol together with the calcium channel blocker diltiazem was shown to have a more substantial beneficial effect than either agent alone [27]. It was argued that this combined effect resulted from the vasodilator action of diltiazem along with the hemodynamic actions of β-blockade. However, it is interesting to note that both drugs have a negative chronotropic action and that when combined, the exercise heart rate was lower than with either agent alone.

From this initial study, the mechanism of the therapeutic action of β-blockade was unclear. The reduction of exercise heart rate was likely involved, but the contribution of the negative inotropic action of β-blockade to the overall efficacy of the drug could not be differentiated. For example, the negative inotropic effect on the outer layers of the post-stenotic region could have reduced metabolic demand there, such that transmural coronary *steal* was lessened. Therefore, further studies were performed to test the importance of heartrate reduction to the beneficial effect of β-adrenoceptor blockade [21]. A similar experimental protocol to that described above was employed, however, in the second run performed after administration of the β-blocker, atrial pacing was begun during the run to prevent the β-blockade-induced bradycardia. Thus, the effect of β-blockade could be observed without its negative chronotropic effect. These studies showed that when exercise heart rate was not reduced, β-blockade no longer had any beneficial effect on regional blood flow (Fig. 4) or contractile function (Fig. 5). In fact, ventricular performance remained significantly impaired (reduced wallthickening in the non-ischemic control areas and depressed LV dP/dt) and ischemic blood flow

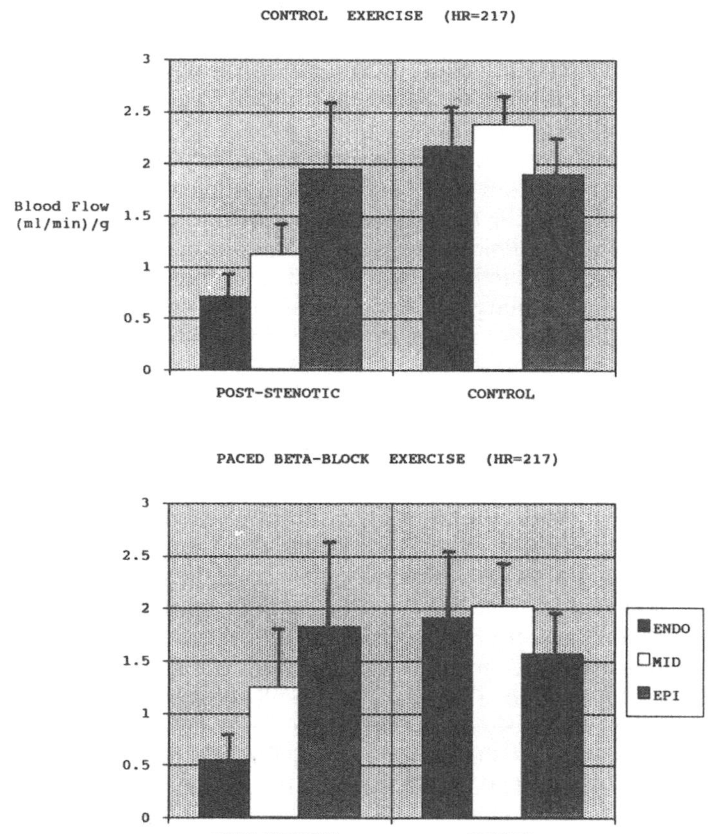

Fig. 4. Atrial pacing was used in a set of studies to prevent the β-blockade-induced bradycardia. When the heart rate was not allowed to decrease after β-blockade, blood flow to the post-stenotic region was no longer improved and tended to be less than that observed in the control run. Therefore, β-blockade without heart rate reduction does not improve post-stenotic blood flow.

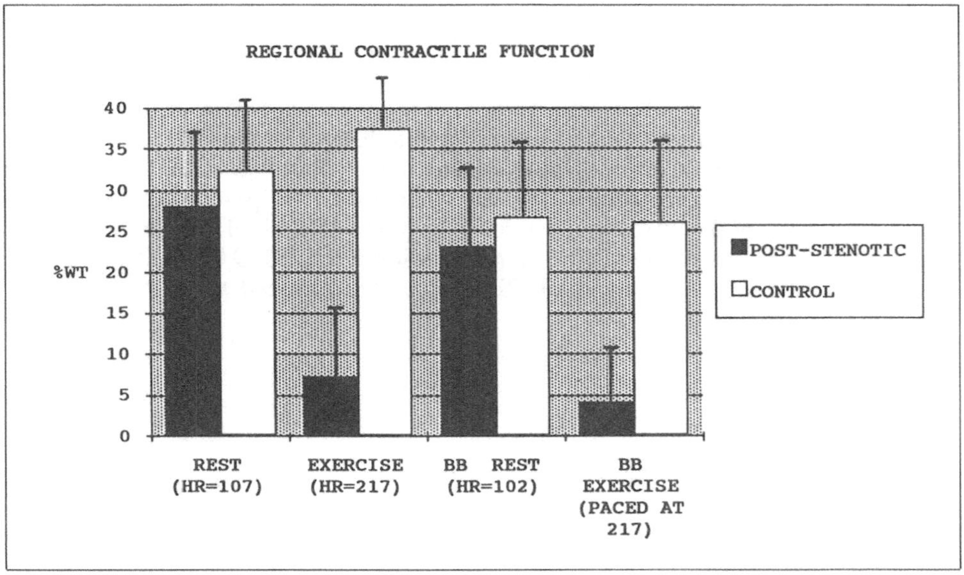

Fig. 5. When heart rate was not allowed to decrease during exercise following β-blockade, post-stenotic regional function was no longer improved in comparison to the control run. Also, there was a depression of function in the control wall.

tended to be further *reduced* compared to the control exercise bout (Fig. 4). This result indicates that the heartrate reduction is essential to the beneficial action of β-blockade during exercise-induced ischemia in this canine model. Additionally, it suggests that the negative inotropic action of β-blockade, by itself, is not advantageous to the acutely ischemic myocardium in terms of either post-stenotic blood flow or contractile function. Thus, a reversal of transmural *steal* by reducing the inotropic state of the outer left ventricular wall did not occur in the absence of heartrate reduction. These results suggest that heartrate reduction achieved *without* concomitant negative inotropism might be advantageous so as to preserve the contractile performance of non-ischemic areas of the heart to better maintain overall cardiac performance.

Treatment of effort angina with a bradycardic agent

Bradycardia is an attractive therapeutic approach for ischemic heart disease due to the unique effect that myocardial contraction has upon its own perfusion, as mentioned above. A reduction of heart rate has been shown recently to have profound effects on regional contractile function and blood flow in acutely ischemic myocardium [7, 17, 18, 25]. These agents are especially appealing in the treatment of effort-induced angina pectoris since it is primarily the tachycardia which induces the ischemia. Thus, reduction of an effort-induced heart rate increase not only lessens the resultant ischemia, but might actually prevent the ischemia from occurring.

The efficacy of the bradycardic agent ULFS 49 CL (Dr. Karl Thomae, Biberach FRG) was therefore studied in the canine model of exercise-induced ischemia described above. A set of original tracings taken from one such study is presented in Fig. 6. During the initial control exercise, heart rate increased from 114 to 230 bpm and severe regional myocardial ischemia occurred with a subendocardial blood flow (measured with radioactive microspheres) in the post-stenotic myocardium of 0.55 (ml/min)/g, as compared to 2.51 (ml/min)/g in a distant, control area (Fig. 7). This was associated with severe regional contractile dysfunction with a reduction in systolic wall thickening from a control value of 23 % (percentage increase in left-ventricular thickness during systole) to only 9 % (Fig. 8). Three hours later, the dogs were run again, following the administration of ULFS 49 CL (1.0 mg/kg, i.v.). Exercise heart rate following ULFS 49 CL was reduced to 139 bpm with a

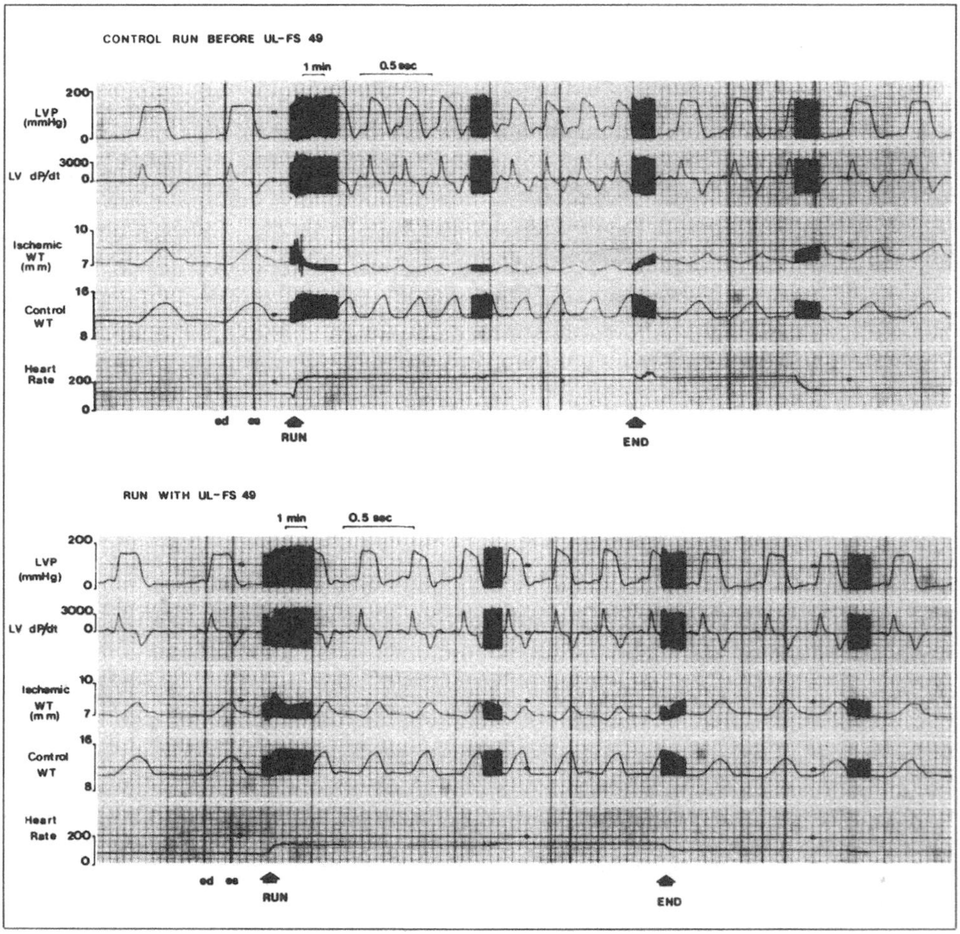

Fig. 6. Original recordings from one study in which ULFS 49 CL was used to reduce exercise heart rate. The parameters recorded were left ventricular pressure (LVP) and its first derivative (LV dP/dt), wall thicknesses in the post-stenotic (IWT) and control walls (CWT), and arterial pressure. In the control run, there is severe regional myocardial dysfunction developing the post-stenotic wall. Following the administration of ULFS 49 CL, exercise produced a significantly lower heart rate and the amount of contractile dysfunction in the post-stenotic region was substantially reduced. Wall-thickening in the control wall was not affected.

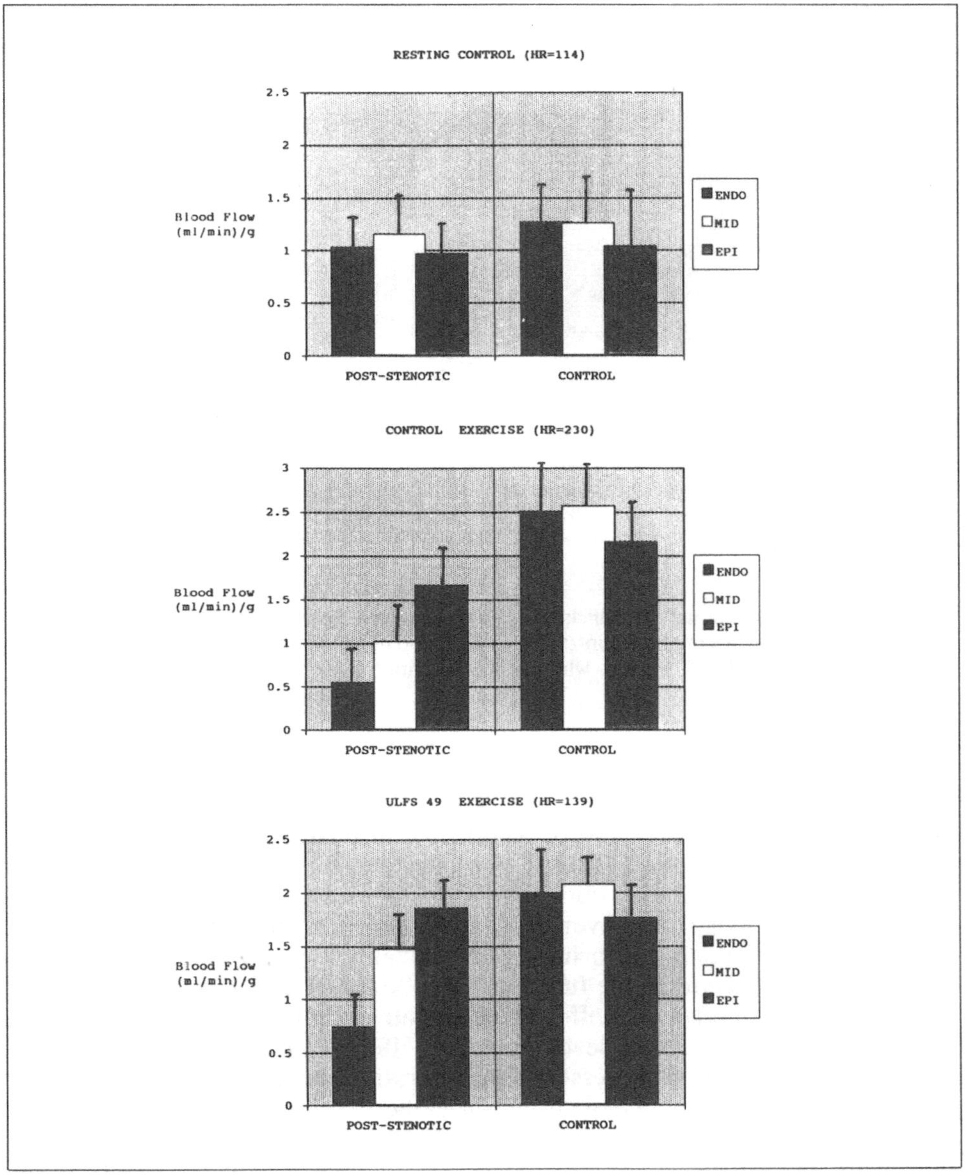

Fig. 7. Summary of blood-flow data during resting conditions, during a control exercise bout, and during exercise following the administration of ULFS 49 CL. The transmural redistribution of blood flow in the post-stenotic region during control exercise was the same as that observed in previous studies. Exercise following ULFS 49 CL produced a greatly reduced heart-rate response and improved blood flow to the post-stenotic subendocardium. Blood flow to the control region was only slightly affected by ULFS 49 CL. Mean ± SD, N = 10.

substantial improvement in the contractile function of the ischemic region to 22 %, a value unchanged from the resting condition (Figs. 6 and 8). There was also a significant improvement in subendocardial blood flow *per minute* (0.55 to 0.75

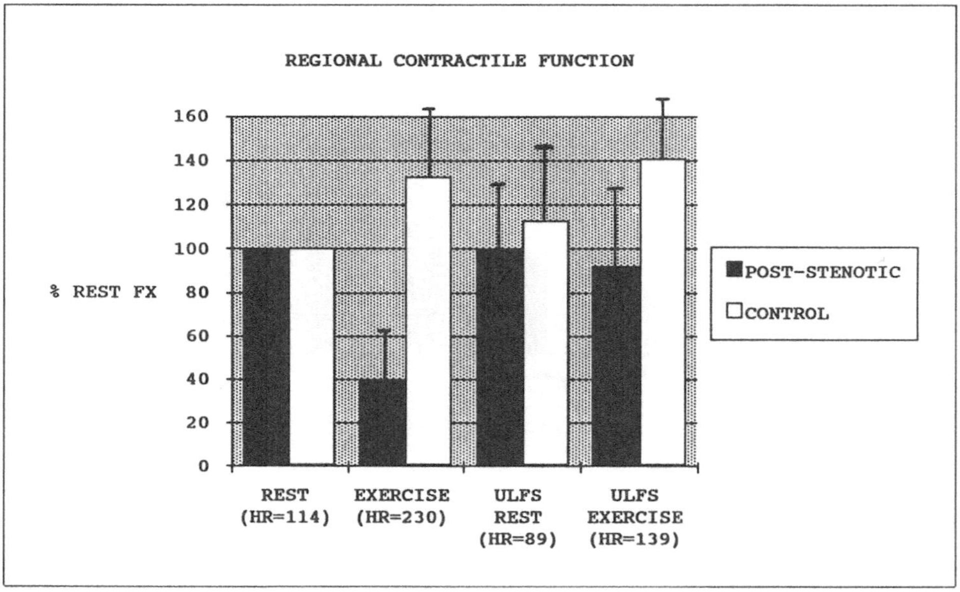

Fig. 8. Summary of regional wall-thickening during exercise before and after administration of ULFS 49 CL. The severe regional contractile dysfunction observed in the post-stenotic region was markedly reduced by ULFS 49 CL, whereas the function in the control region was unaffected.

(ml/min)/g) (Fig. 7). Although the increase in regional wall thickening appears to be considerably larger than the observed increase in blood flow, it must be remembered that it is the ratio of blood flow to heart rate which best predicts regional contractile function. Thus, if one calculates the amount of blood flow *per beat* as a way of incorporating both blood flow and heart rate changes, the increase following ULFS 49 CL was over two-fold (blood flow increased and heart rate decreased, therefore the ratio improved substantially) and consistent with the increase in regional contractile function. Despite the profound exercise bradycardia, the other hemodynamic effects were relatively minor. Peak leftventricular pressure and rate of pressure development (LV dP/dt) were unaffected. However, end-diastolic leftventricular pressure was significantly increased during the run with reduced heart rate. (This increase in end-diastolic pressure may have acted to offset the expected decrease in leftventricular dP/dt due to a negative force-frequency effect with the heartrate reduction.) The approximately 90 bpm reduction in heart rate achieved in the exercising dog is much larger than one would anticipate in clinical usage. Thus, the elevated end-diastolic left-ventricular pressure may not be apparent with more modest heart-rate reductions. It is important to note that regional contractile function in the control, non-ischemic myocardium was not impaired by ULFS 49 CL, and that this lack of effect on the non-ischemic myocardium likely plays a role in the maintenance of overall left-ventricular function. Thus, the prevention of exercise-induced tachycardia through the use of the bradycardic agent ULFS 49 CL improved the ischemic myocardial blood flow and function to a far greater extent than that achieved through β-blockade, and without the additional negative inotropism associated with the use of β-blockers.

These impressive results have been confirmed by an independent study using a slightly different experimental model [35].

Conclusions

It must be emphasized that the application of experimental results to the clinical setting should be done with caution. The canine experimental model used has only a single-vessel stenosis, and collateral development in the dog is often extensive, whereas human coronary disease involves multiple vessels and collateral coronary circulation may be sparse. Nevertheless, the efficacy of heart-rate reduction for the treatment of, or *prevention* of exercise-induced ischemia is reliant upon fundamental mechanisms in the pathophysiological genesis of effort angina pectoris. From the perspective of the experimental approach employed, reduction of heart rate through the use of a bradycardic agent has provided the single-most effective intervention for the reduction of regional myocardial ischemia and improvement of contractile function during exercise-induced ischemia [20]. A similarly large improvement in regional blood flow and function has only been observed through the combined use of a β-blocker, calcium antagonist, and a nitrate [19]. However, even in this combined therapy, heart-rate reduction was likely a major contributor to the lessened exercise-induced ischemia.

References

1. Ball RM, Bache RJ (1976) Distribution of myocardial blood flow in the exercising dog with restricted coronary artery inflow. Circ Res 38: 60–66
2. Ball RM, Bache RJ, Cobb FR, Greenfield Jr JC (1975) Regional myocardial blood flow during graded treadmill exercise in the dog. J Clin Invest 55: 43–49
3. Bache RJ, Cobb FR (1977) Effect of maximal coronary vasodilation on transmural myocardial perfusion during tachycardia in the awake dog. Circ Res 41: 648–653
4. Bassenge E, Kucharczyk M, Holtz J, Stoian D (1972) Treadmill exercise in dogs under beta-adrenergic blockade: adaptation of coronary and systemic hemodynamics. Pfluegers Arch 332: 40–55
5. Becker L (1976) Effect of tachycardia on left ventricular blood flow distribution during coronary occlusion. Am J Physiol 230: 1072–1077
6. Berdeaux A, Garnier M, Boissier JR, Giudicelli JF (1979) The role of beta-adrenoceptors in coronary blood flow distribution in normal and ischemic canine myocardium. Eur J Pharmacol 53: 261–271
7. Buck JD, Hardman HF, Warltier DC, Gross GJ (1981) Changes in ischemic blood flow distribution and dynamic severity of a coronary stenosis induced by beta blockade in the canine heart. Circulation 64: 708–715
8. Canty JM (1988) Coronary pressure-function and steady-state pressure-flow relations during autoregulation in the unanesthetized dog. Circ Res 63: 821–836
9. Domenech RJ, de la Prida JM (1975) Mechanical effects of heart contraction on coronary flow. Cardiovasc Res 9: 509–514
10. Epstein SE, Braunwald E (1966) Beta-adrenergic receptors blocking drugs. Mechanisms of action and clinical applications. N Engl J Med 275: 1106–1112
11. Gallagher KP, Folts JD, Shebuski RJ, Rankin JHG, Rowe GG (1980) Subepicardial vasodilator reserve in the presence of critical coronary stenosis in dogs. Am J Cardiol 46: 67–73

12. Gallagher KP, Matsuzaki M, Koziol JA, Kemper WS, Ross Jr J (1984) Regional myocardial perfusion and wall thickening during ischemia in conscious dogs. Am J Physiol 247: H727–H738
13. Gallagher KP, Matsuzaki M, Osakada G, Kemper WS, Ross Jr J (1983) Effect of exercise on the relationship betwen myocardial blood flow and systolic wall thickening in dogs with acute coronary stenosis. Circ Res 52: 716–729
14. Gallagher KP, Osakada G, Matsuzaki M, Kemper WS, Ross Jr J (1982) Myocardial blood flow and function with critical coronary stenosis in exercising dogs. Am J Physiol 243: H698–H707
15. Garcia-Dorado D, Theroux P, Elizaya J, Galiñanes M, Solares J, Riesgo M, Gomez MJ, Garcia-Dorado A, Aviles Ff (1987) Myocardial reperfusion in the pig heart model: infarct size and duration of coronary occlusion. Cardiovas Res 21: 537–544
16. Gregg DE (1974) The natural history of coronary collateral development. Circ Res 35: 335–344
17. Gross GJ, Dämmgen JW (1987) Effect of the new specific bradycardic agent AQ-A 39 (falipamil) on coronary collateral blood flow in dogs. J Cardiovasc Pharmacol 10: 123–127
18. Gross GJ, Lamping KG, Warltier DC, Hardman HF (1984) Effects of three bradycardiac drugs on regional myocardial blood flow and function in areas distal to a total or partial coronary occlusion in dogs. Circulation 69: 391–399
19. Guth BD, Tajimi T, Seitelberger R, Lee JD, Matsuzaki M, Ross Jr J (1986) Experimental exercise-induced ischemia: drug therapy can eliminate regional dysfunction and oxygen supply-demand imbalance. J Am Coll Cardiol 7: 1036–1046
20. Guth BD, Heusch G, Seitelberger R, Ross Jr J (1987) Elimination of exercise-induced regional myocardial dysfunction by a bradycardic agent in dogs with chronic coronary stenosis. Circulation 75: 661–669
21. Guth BD, Heusch G, Seitelberger R, Ross Jr J (1987) Mechanism of beneficial effect of beta-adrenergic blockade on exercise-induced myocardial ischemia in conscious dogs. Circ Res 60: 738–746
22. Guth BD, Schulz R, Thaulow E (1991) Intervertricular redistribution of myocardial blood flow during metabolic vasodilation. Pflügers Arch 417: 485–492
23. Heusch G, Schulte W, Rüddel H, Neus H (1981) Laerm und vegetatives Nervensystem. Therapiewoche 31: 33–36
24. Hjalmarson A (1984) The Göteborg metoprolol trial in acute myocardial infarction. Am J Cardiol 53 Suppl.: 1D
25. Indolfi C, Guth BD, Miura T, Miyazaki S, Schulz R, Ross Jr J (1989) Mechanisms of improved ischemic regional dysfunction by bradycardia. Studies on ULFS 49 CL in swine. Circulation 80: 983–993
26. Matsuzaki M, Gallagher KP, Patritti J, Tajimi T, Kemper WS, White FC, Ross Jr J (1984) Effects of a calcium-entry blocker (diltiazem) on regional myocardial flow and function during exercise in conscious dogs. Circulation 69: 801–814
27. Matsuzaki M, Guth BD, Tajimi T, Kemper WS, Ross Jr J (1985) Effects of the combination of diltiazem and atenolol on exercise-induced regional myocardial ischemia in conscious dogs. Circulation 72: 233–243
28. Matsuzaki M, Patritti J, Tajimi T, Miller M, Kemper WS, Ross Jr J (1984) Effects of β-blockade on regional myocardial flow and function during exercise. Am J Physiol 247: H52–H60
29. Murakami H, Kim S-J, Downey HF (1989) Persistent right coronary flow reserve at low perfusion pressure. Am J Physiol 256: H1176–H1184
30. Neill WA, Oxendine JM, Phelps NC, Anderson RP (1975) Subendocardial ischemia provoked by tachycardia in conscious dogs with coronary stenosis. Am J Cardiol 35: 30–36
31. Neill WA, Phelps NC, Oxendine JM, Mahler DJ, Sim DN (1973) Effect of heart rate on coronary blood flow distribution in dogs. Am J Cardiol 32: 306–312
32. Pantely GA, Bristow JD, Swenson LJ, Ladley HD, Johnson WE, Anselone CG (1985) Incomplete coronary vasodilation during myocardial ischemia in swine. Am J Physiol 249: H638–H647

33. Pasyk S, Flameng W, Wüsten B, Schaper W (1976) Influence of tachycardia on regional myocardial flow in chronic experimental coronary occlusion. Basic Res Cardiol 71: 243–251
34. Pitt B, Gregg DE (1968) Coronary hemodynamic effects of increasing ventricular rate in the unanesthetized dog. Circ Res 22: 753–761
35. Raberger G, Krumpl G, Schneider W (1987) Effects of bradycardic agent ULFS 49 CL on exercise-induced regional contractile dysfunction in dogs. Int J Cardiol 14: 343–354
36. Raff WK, Kosche F, Lochner W (1971) Herzfrequenz und extravasale Komponente des Coronarwiderstandes. Pfluegers Arch 323: 241–249
37. Ross J Jr (1989) Mechanism of regional ischemia and antianginal drug action during exercise. Prog Cardiovasc Dis 31: 455–466
38. Santamore WP, Bove AA, Carey RA (1982) Tachycardia induced reduction in coronary blood flow distal to a stenosis. Int J Cardiol 2: 23–37
39. Sasayama S, Franklin D, Ross Jr J, Kemper WS, McKown D (1976) Dynamic changes in left ventricular wall thickness and their use in analyzing cardiac function in the conscious dogs. Am J Cardiol 38: 870–879
40. Schulz R, Miyazaki S, Miller M, Thaulow E, Heusch G, Ross J Jr, Guth BD (1989) Consequences of regional inotropic stimulation of ischemic myocardium on regional myocardial blood flow and function in anesthetized swine. Circ Res 64: 1116–1126
41. Stein PD, Marzilli M, Sabbah HN, Lee T (1980) Systolic and diastolic pressure gradients within the left ventricular wall. Am J Physiol 238: H625–H630
42. Thuillez C, Berdeaux A, Bonhenry C, Duhaye P, Guidicelli JF (1983) Effects of propranol on regional myocardial blood flow and function during severe coronary stenosis in dogs. Eur J Pharmacol 92: 171–179
43. Vatner SF (1980) Correlation between acute reductions in myocardial blood flow and function in conscious dogs. Circ Res 47: 201–207
44. Waagstein F, Hjalmarson AC (1976) Double-blind study of the effect of cardioselective beta-blockade on chest pain in acute myocardial infarction. Acta Med Scand 587 Suppl.: 201–208

Author's address:
Brian D. Guth, Ph. D.,
Pharmakologie E, J81
Dr. Karl Thomae, GmbH
Postfach 1755
D-7950 Biberach an der Riß

Electrophysiological effects of ULFS 49 CL

K. Seidl, B. Hauer, W. Lengfelder, J. Senges

Klinikum Ludwigshafen

Introduction

Pharmacologically, a decrease in sinus heart rate can be achieved by several means: indirectly, via inhibition of the autonomic nervous system, and directly at the pacemaker cells of the atrial sinus node. The term "Specific Bradycardic Agents" has been proposed for drugs which directly decrease the sinus rate in doses or concentrations smaller than are necessary to elicit other pharmacological effects [1, 7, 9, 10, 13]. ULFS 49 CL is such a new, specific, negative chronotropic agent which directly decreases the spontaneous heart rate by slowing the diastolic depolarization of the pacemaker cells in the sinu-atrial node [6, 8, 11].

Since other agents that also reduce the heart rate (β-blocker, calcium antagonists) produce a prolongation of the cardiac conduction times [4, 12], the effect of ULFS 49 CL on cardiac conduction was investigated in this study.

The purpose of the study was to evaluate the effects of ULFS 49 CL on the electrophysiologic parameters in man, and to evaluate its short-term tolerability.

Patient characteristics

The study was performed as a double-blind, randomized, placebo-controlled group comparison. Twenty-four patients who gave their informed consent were randomly

Table 1. Patient characteristics (n = 22)

	Placebo (n = 11)	ULFS 49 CL (n = 11)
Age (year)	56 ± 15	52 ± 8
Sex	f = 4	f = 2
	m = 7	m = 9
CHD	4	6
Cardiomyopathy	0	1
Mitral prolapse	0	1
No organic heart disease	7	3

allocated to either ULFS 49 CL or placebo, 22 of whom were analyzed. There were 16 men and six women with a mean age of 54 + 12 years. Ten patients had a coronary heart disease, one patient had a cardiomyopathy, one had a mitral valve prolapse, the remaining 10 patients did not have any organic heart disease (Table 1).

The indication for invasive electrophysiologic study was unexplained syncope in 19 patients; three patients suffered from palpitations and presyncope (Table 2).

Table 2. Indications for electrophysiologic study

(n = 11)	Placebo (n = 11)	ULFS 49 CL
Syncope	8	11
Palpitation and Presnycope	3	0

The clinical characteristics of both groups were comparable regarding age, sex, underlying heart disease, and regarding the indication for the electropysiologic study.

The baseline characteristics are distributed homogeneously and do not differ significantly between the two treatment groups.

Method (Fig. 1)

In all patients an electrophysiologic study with intracardiac recording and programmed stimulation was performed. Three catheters were advanced from the

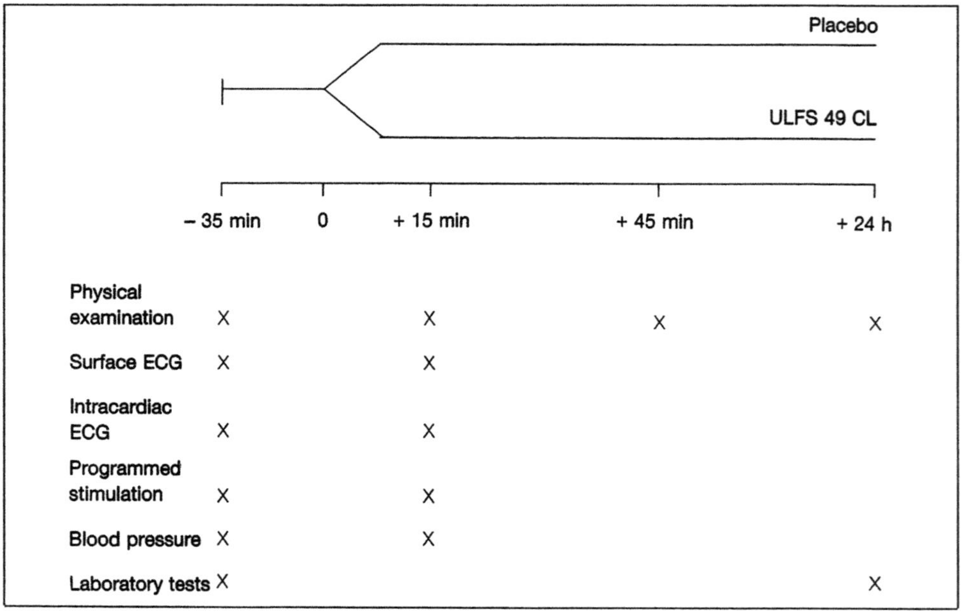

Fig. 1. Methods

right femoral vein into the right heart. A quadripolar catheter was placed in the high right atrium. The distal pair of electrodes was used for stimulation, the proximal pair for sensing. The potentials of the His-bundle were recorded with a bipolar catheter. A quadripolar catheter was positioned in the apex of the right ventricle. All stimulations were performed with the two-fold diastolic threshold current.

The study medication was identical in appearance. All medication with potential cardiac and antiarrhytmic effects were discontinued at least 5 half-lives-times. After injection of 5 mg (which is 5 ml trial medication) a maintenance infusion of 5 mg over 45 min followed in order to keep the plasma levels constant.

Before and within 15 min after the bolus-injection the following investigations were performed: a physical examination, a surface ECG, intracardiac ECG, programmed stimulation, blood-pressure measurement, and laboratory tests. A physical examination was done again after 45 min and 24 h later. Laboratory tests were again taken 24h later.

The following electrophysiologic parameters were measured at sinus rhythm or at atrial (right ventricular) stimulation with 550 ms cycle length: spontaneous sinus node cycle length (S-CL), sinus node recovery time (SNRT), rate corrected sinus node recovery time (CSNRT), and conduction times from low right atrium to the His-bundle (AH), and from the His-bundle to the depolarization of the septum (HV). The refractory periods of the atrioventricular node (ERP-AV) were determined by the extrastimuli technique at a paced atrial cycle lenght of 550 ms, and the effective refractory period of the right ventricle (ERP-RV) at a paced ventricular cycle length of 550 ms.

All recordings were performed with a Mingograf (Siemens Elema) at a paper speed of 50 mm/s and 100 mm/s.

The baseline data were compared between the groups by analysis of variance. The *t*-test for paired observations was used to compare the values before and after treatment. Analysis of variance of differences was used to compare the differences after/before between the two treatment groups; $p < 0.05$ was considered statistically significant. All results are expressed as means (X) ± SD.

Results

All measured ECG-intervals (PQ, QRS, QTc) were comparable at baseline and remained unchanged during treatment with the study medication. The changes after/before did not differ between the groups (Fig. 2).

The sinus cycle length was comparable between the treatment groups at baseline, but the changes after/before were significantly different between both treatment groups. The difference of changes was 95 ms (Fig. 3).

Baseline sinus node recovery time was comparable between both groups. It remained unchanged after treatment with placebo and was statistically significant increased after ULFS 49 CL. However, comparing the rate corrected sinus node recovery time no statistically significant change, neither within nor between the treatment groups, could be detected (Fig. 3).

AH intervals remained unchanged and no group difference of changes appeared (Fig. 4).

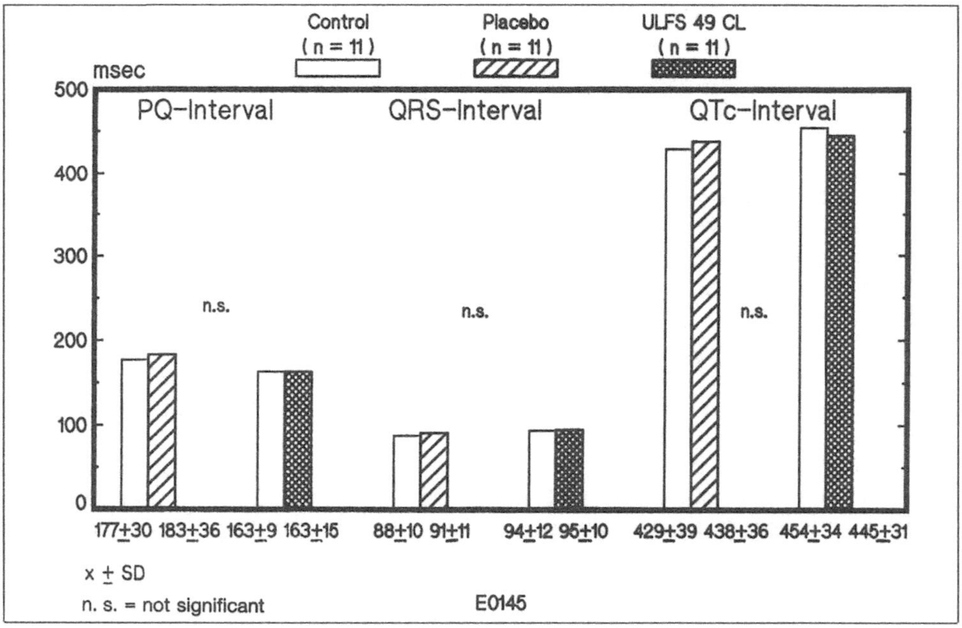

Fig. 2. Effect on electrocardiographic parameters. Mean values before and after treatment. The analysis of variance of differences was used to compare the differences after/before between the two treatment groups.

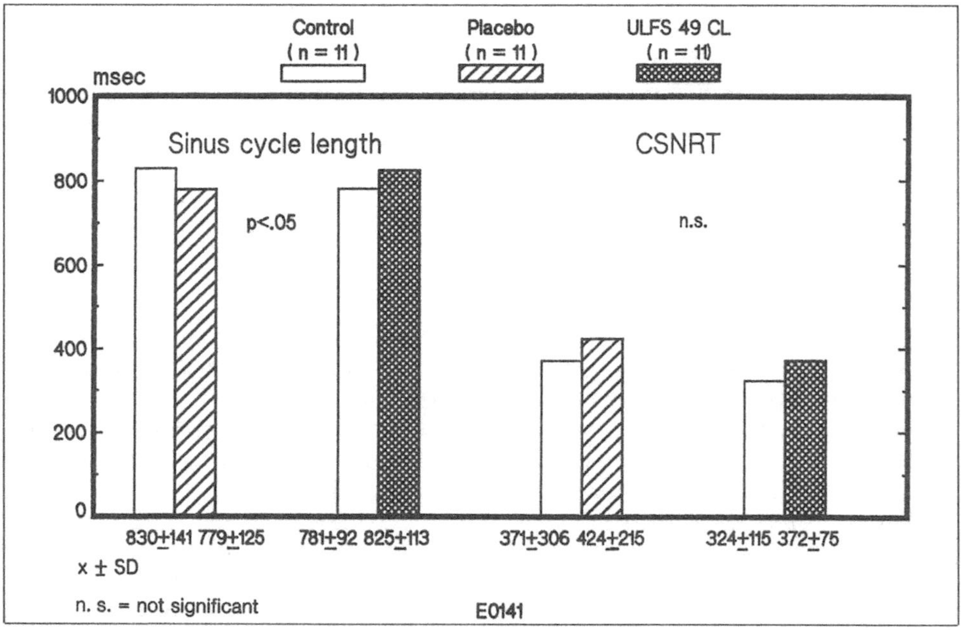

Fig. 3. Effect on sinus cycle length and corrected sinus node recovery time (CSNRT). Mean values before and after treatment. The analysis of variance of differences was used to compare the differences after/before between the two treatment groups.

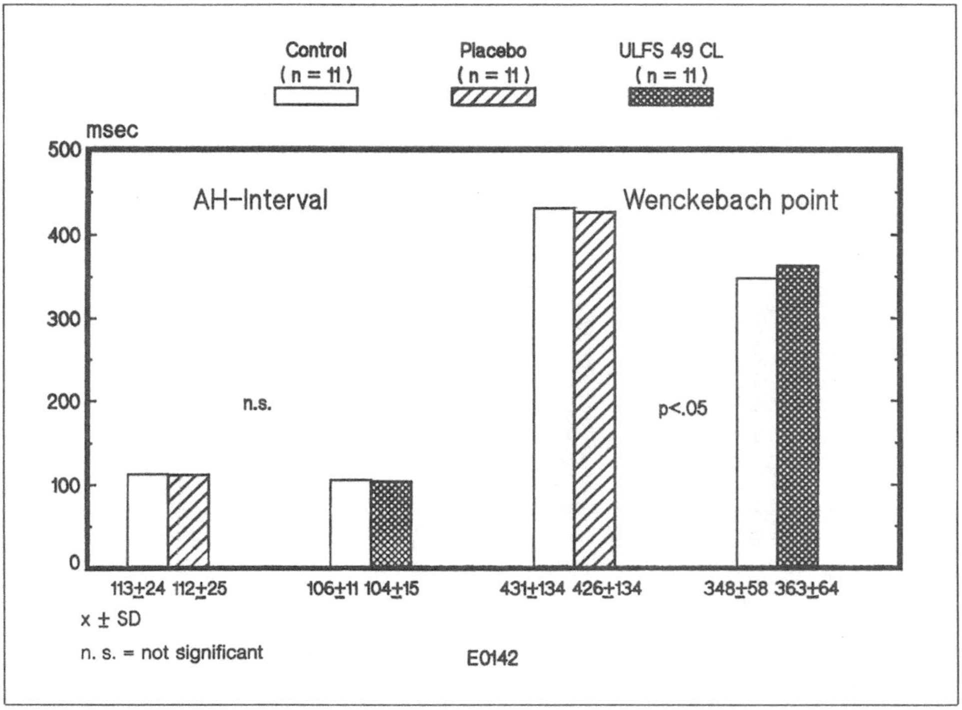

Fig. 4. Effects on AH-interval and Wenckebach point. Mean values before and after treatment. The analysis of variance of differences was used to compare the differences after/before between the two treatment groups.

The Wenckebach- point was slightly, but not significantly reduced in the placebo group and was slightly increased in the ULFS 49 CL group, resulting in a significant group difference of changes (Fig. 4).

Two patients in each treatment group were found to have a pathological HV-interval at baseline. Comparing the values before and after treatment with the study medication, placebo did not alter the HV-interval to a statistically significant degree. ULFS 49 CL increased the HV-interval by 10 % ($p < 0.05$) with a statistically significant group difference of 7 ms (Fig. 5).

When only the patients with non-pathological baseline HV-intervals are compared, neither placebo nor ULFS 49 CL altered the parameters to a statistically significant degree, and no group difference of changes appeared (Fig. 5).

Baseline ERP-AV and ERP-RV were comparable between both treatment groups and did not change after treatment, neither within nor between the groups (Fig. 6).

Both systolic and diastolic blood pressure were comparable at baseline and neither of them was altered by the study medication.

In this study, no side effects were observed after short term i.v. administration in either treatment group.

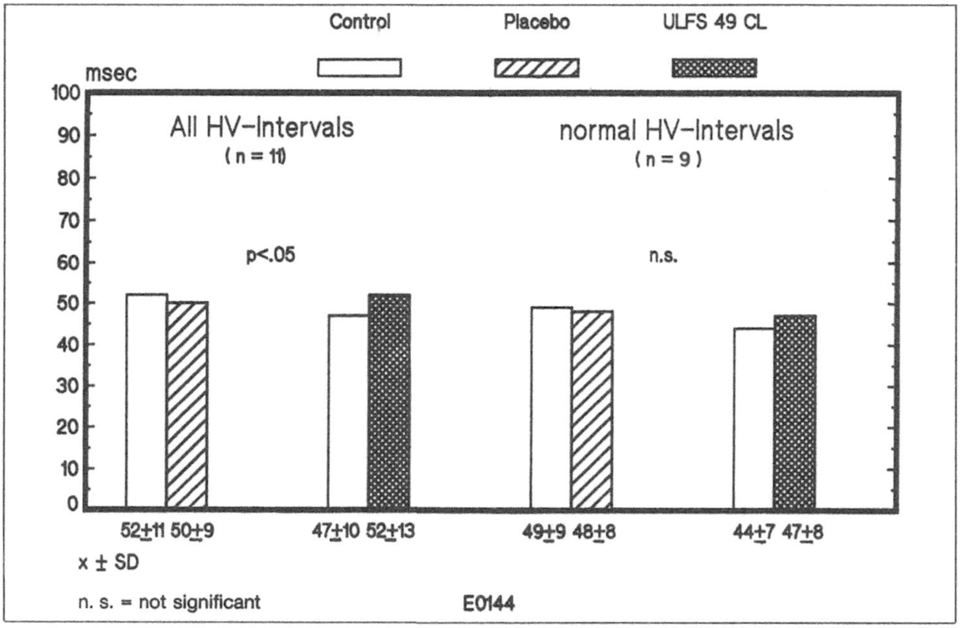

Fig. 5. Effects of the HV-interval. Mean values before and after treatment. The analysis of variance of differences was used to compare the differences after/before between the two treatment groups.

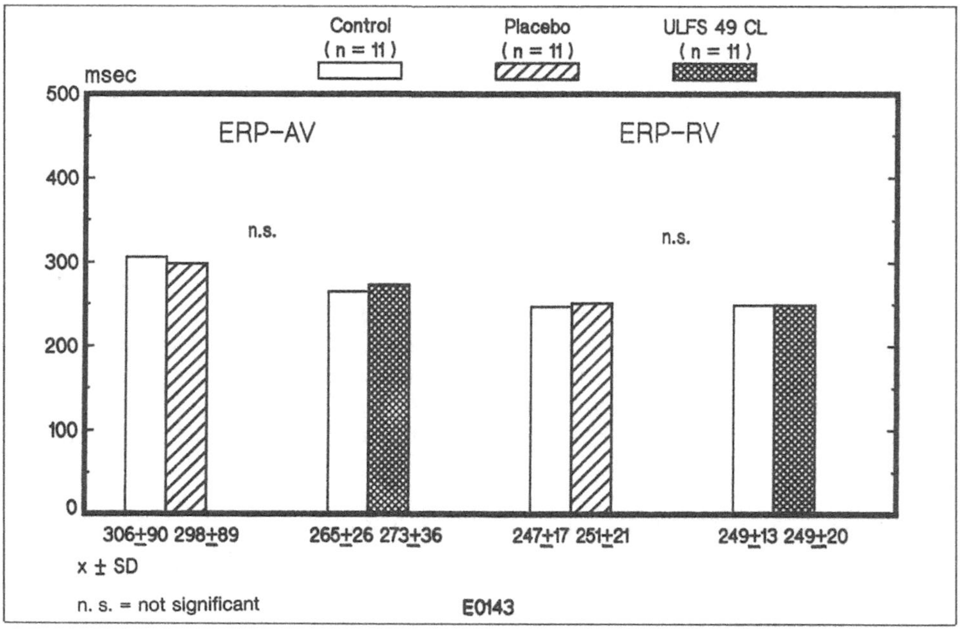

Fig. 6. Effects of the effective refractory periods of the AV-node (ERP-AV) and right ventricle (ERP-RV). Mean values before and after treatment. The analysis of variance of differences was used to compare the differences after/before between the two treatment groups.

Discussion

In cases of coronary artery disease a decrease in myocardial oxygen consumption is a desired therapeutic measure. It may be achieved by decreasing myocardial contractility, decreasing tension development or decreasing heart rate. The decrease in sinus heart rate seems the most disirable approach to the problem, provided that it is due to a prolongation of the diastolic period, the time-span which allows perfusion of the myocardium.

The term "Specific Bradycardic Agents" has been proposed for drugs including a certain haemodynamic pattern, namely a decrease in sinus heart rate when in doses or concentrations smaller than those necessary to elicit other pharmacological effects [7, 10, 13].

Several animal studies have shown a specific negative chronotopic effect on the sinu-atrial node of ULFS 49 CL. In these studies, ULFS 49 CL caused a reversible bradycardia by a reduction of the rate of diastolic depolarization, and an increase in the duration of the last part of the repolarization [1, 5, 14].

Since other agents that also reduce the heart rate (β-blockers, calciumantagonists of the verapamil type) produce a prolongation of the cardiac conduction times (4, 12), the effect of ULFS 49 CL on conduction times was investigated in man in the present study.

The results demonstrate that the administration of 10 mg ULFS 49 CL i.v. led to a decrease of the heart rate by mean difference of 7 bpm ($p < 0.05$) relative to placebo.

The rate-corrected sinus node recovery time, the AH-interval, the effective refractory periods of the AV-node and the right ventricle, and the ventriculo-atrial conduction time remained unaltered.

The Wenckebach-point, i.e., the longest atrial cycle length where 1:1 stimulus propagation occurs was slightly prolonged by 15 ms in the ULFS 49 CL group and was reduced by 5 ms in the placebo group, resulting in a statistically significant group difference ($p < 0.05$). If the Wenckebach-point was calculated in bpm, this would mean a reduction from 172 bpm to 165 bpm, where an AV-block occurred. This is considered as being clinically not relevant.

Two patients in each treatment group demonstrated a pathological HV-interval at baseline. When these four patients remained in the evaluation, ULFS 49 CL prolonged the HV-interval relative to placebo by 7 ms ($p < 0.05$). When only the patients with non pathological baseline values were evaluated, ULFS 49 CL did not alter the HV-intervals in comparison to placebo.

Conclusion

1) ULFS 49 CL, in low doses, results in a negative chronotropic effect on the sinus node in humans.
2) ULFS 49 CL does not exert additional electrophysiological effects in patients without disturbance of the AV-conduction.
3) However, in patients with pathological HV-interval an increase of the HV-interval results after intravenous administration of ULFS 49 CL.
4) Side-effects did not occur during i.v. administration.

The results suggest that ULFS 49 CL does not alter the intracardial conduction times in patients with non-pathological baseline values. In patients with prolonged HV-interval, administration of ULFS 49 CL results in a further prolongation. In order to exclude clinical, serious effects on an impaired AV-conduction system further investigations are needed.

References

1. Bouman LN, Ginneken A van, Opthof T, Duivenvoorden JJ (1986) Electrophysiology of sinoatrial node and the action of specific bradycardic agents (SBA), a novel approach to cardiac physiology and therapy. International workshop at the Ernst Boehringer Institut, Bender u. Co
2. Buckberg GD, Fixler DE, Archie JP, Hoffman JIE (1972) Experimental subendocardial ischemia in dogs with normal coronary arteries. Circ Res, 30: 67–81
3. Buckberg GD, Fixler DE, Archie JP, Henney RP, Hoffman JIE (1975) Variable effects of heart rate on phasic and regional left ventricular muscle blood flow in anesthetized dogs. Cardiovasc Res 9: 1–11
4. Connoly ME, Kersting F, Dollery CT (1976) The clinical pharmacology of beta-adrenergic blocking drugs. Prog Cardiovasc Dis 19: 203–49
5. Dämmgen JW, Lamping KA, Gross GJ (1985) Action of two new bradycardic agents, AQ-AH 208 and ULFS 49, on ischemic myocardial perfusion and function. J Cardiovasc Pharmacol 7: 71–79
6. Gruber R, Lumper G, Zilberszac A, Heistracher P (1983) Effects of ULFS 49 CL on the action potential of the guinea-pig heart. Naunyn-Schmiedeberg's Arch. Pharmacol. 324, R 32
7. Heistracher P (1986) Specific bradycardic agents: Introduction; specific bradycardic agents, a novel approach to cardiac physiology and therapy. International workshop at the Ernst-Boehringer-Institut, Bender u. Co
8. Kobinger W, Lillie C (1984a) Cardiovascular characterization of ULFS 49 CL, a new "specific bradycardic agent". Eur. J. Pharmacol. 104: 9–18
9. Kobinger W, Lillie C (1984b) New Drugs Annual: Cardiovascular Drugs, Vol. 2, Chapter 10, 193–210, ed. by Alexander Scriabine, Raven Press, New York
10. Kobinger W (1985) Specific bradycardic agents, a new approach to therapy in angina pectoris? Prog Pharmacol 5 (3), 89–100
11. Lillie C, Kobinger W (1983) Cardiovascular actions of ULFS 49, a new "specific bradycardic agent", Naunyn-Schmiedeberg's Arch. Pharmacol. 324, R 33
12. Mc Allister RG Jr. (1982) Clinical pharmacology of slow channel calcium blocking agents. Prog Cardiovasc Dis 25: 83–102
13. Reiffen M (1985) Specific bradycardic agents- a new principle in coronary heart disease 189th ACS National Meeting, American Chemical Society, Division of Medical Chemistry Abstr 41
14. Senges Rizos I, Brachmann J, Anders G, Jauerning R, Hamman H-D, Kübler W (1983) Effect of nifedipine and AQ-A39 on the sinoatrial and atrioventricular nodes of the rabbit and their antiarrhythmic action on atrioventricular nodal reentrant tachycardia. Cardiovasc Res 17: 132–144
15. Sonnenblick EH; Skeleton CL (1971) Oxygen consumption of the heart: Physiological principles and clinical implications. Mod concepts Cardiovasc Dis 40, 9–16

Authors' address:
Dr. K. Seidl,
Klinikum Ludwigshafen,
6700 Ludwigshafen/Rhein, FRG

Antiischemic, antianginal, and hemodynamic effects of ULFS 49 CL (a new heart-rate-reducing agent) in patients with angiographically proven CAD

H. F. Pitschner[1], E. Muno[1], F. Vens-Cappel[1], B. Schulte[1], M. Schlepper[1], V. de Moura-Sieber[2], W. Baiker[3]

[1] Kerckhoff-Klinik of the Max-Planck Society, Bad Nauheim, FRG; [2] Boehringer Ingelheim, Dept. of Medicine, Cardiology, Ingelheim, FRG; [3] Dr. Karl Thomae GmbH, Dept. of Medicine, Cardiology, Biberach, FRG

Introduction

ULFS 49 CL, a so-called sinus node inhibitor, does not affect β-adrenergic or muscarinic receptors at therapeutical plasma concentrations in man. The compound's underlying mechanism of action to decrease heart rate can be explained by an inhibition of the i_f-current, which seems to be responsible for the spontaneous depolarization of the pacemaker cells in the sino-atrial node [1, 2]. Like β-blockers, the substance is expected to produce a reduction in heart rate. Through this mechanism ULFS 49 CL may result in antianginal and/or antiischemic efficacy in patients with angina pectoris. At present, no data are available on its antiischemic potential. The aim of the present multicenter trial was to investigate the antianginal, antiischemic, and hemodynamic effects of ULFS 49 CL, a new heart-rate-reducing compound, in patients with stable angina pectoris.

Methods

The trial was designed as a randomized, double-blind, placebo-controlled group comparison of 2.5 mg and 5 mg ULFS 49 CL. Patients were recruited from eight study centers in the Federal Republic of Germany (West). The trial protocol was approved by the Freiburger Ethics Committee, Freiburg, and patients gave their informed consent according to the revised Declaration of Helsinki.

Inclusion criteria

Only patients with stable angina pectoris and angiographically proven coronary artery disease with a stenosis of at least 60 % in at least one main coronary artery were included in the study. Patients had to be in sinus rhythm. They were excluded from entry into the study if clinical signs of cardiac insufficiency or a history of myocardial infarction with an EF < 50 % were present. Also, patients with variant or unstable angina pectoris were excluded. An ST-segment depression of at least 0.1 mV under exercise had to be demonstrable in order to prove ischemic origin of the anginal pain. Not allowed were patients with clinical signs of atherosclerosis of other organ systems, especially patients with claudicatio intermittens. Moreover patients with rhythm disorders, with obstructive pulmonary disease or with hematological diseases were also excluded. The age limits were 40 to 75 years and patients should be of normal weight (Broca index between –20 % and +20 %). All cardiovascular drugs had to be withdrawn at least five half-life times before start of the study. Administration of short-acting nitrates was allowed, for relief of anginal attacks.

Study protocol

Exercise tests were performed in the supine position with a bicycle ergometer. Prior to the first exercise test on the first study day (on which the individual ergometry protocol was defined), patients had to rest in supine position for 15 min. The initial load of 25 watts was increased in steps of 25 watts every 5 min. Criteria for termination of exercise were onset of moderate anginal pain, ST-segment depression of more than 0.4 mV in leads III, V_2, V_4, or V_6, systolic blood pressure >110 mmHg, or a mean pulmonary artery pressure >40 mmHg.

On the second study day the exercise protocol was repeated with a starting load of 25 watts less than the maximal load reached on the first day. A balloon-tipped Swan-Ganz catheter was placed in the pulmonary artery for measurement of pulmonary capillary pressure (PCP), pulmonary artery pressure (PAP), right atrial pressure (RAP), and cardiac output. After 15 min rest the control exercise test was performed, followed by a recreation phase of at least 60 min. The hemodynamic parameters including heart rate and blood pressure were recorded at 5, 10, and 15 min of exercise. Repeat measurements were performed 10, 30, and 60 min after termination of exercise. After the resting heart rate had returned to control values the study medication (placebo, 2.5 mg or 5.0 mg ULFS 49 CL) was injected intravenously over 5 min. 15 min after injection the study parameters were recorded at rest and at exercise under the same conditions as the control test.

Plasma samples were obtained from the patients 15 min after injection and stored at –20 °C until measurement by HPLC.

Statistical evaluation

To ensure that the calculated treatment effects were not the result of differences between trial centers and age groups, they were tested as excess over trial center and age group effects. As method, the oneway analysis of variance by treatment (nominal) and two-/three-way ANOVA by trial center, age group and treatment (nominal) were used. Between both methods the p-values differed only slightly; the differences between both methods were much smaller than the differences between the first method and the consideration of ordered groups. Therefore, the p-values reported here are the realistic ones, although interaction might be possible [3, 4]. All values are given as mean or mean ± standard deviation (SD). The levels of significance were defined as $p < 0.05$. A value of $p < 0.05$ is indicated by *, $p < 0.01$

Table 1. Summary of hemodynamic results

Parameter (dim.)	Gr.	At rest							During exercise, last comp. values						
		Control	Placebo or ULFS 49 CL	Chg. %	Sign. (A)	Sign. (B)			Control	Placebo or ULFS 49 CL	Chg. %	Sign. (A)	Sign. (B)		
						gr.0	gr.1	gr.2					gr.0	gr.1	gr.2
Heart rate (b/min)	0	72 ± 12	73 ± 12	1					112 ± 15	114 ± 15	2	*		***	***
	1	70 ± 12	68 ± 11	–3					109 ± 19	104 ± 19	–5	***			
	2	70 ± 8	68 ± 8	–4	*				107 ± 16	102 ± 15	–5	***			
Blood pressure															
Syst. (mmHg)	0	138 ± 21	140 ± 19	2					174 ± 23	177 ± 23	2				
	1	137 ± 16	136 ± 16	–1					173 ± 23	169 ± 20	–2				
	2	137 ± 16	134 ± 16	–3	*				168 ± 22	168 ± 23	0				
Diast. (mmHg)	0	84 ± 8	86 ± 10	2					100 ± 12	100 ± 10	0				
	1	84 ± 9	85 ± 10	1					96 ± 11	96 ± 12	0				
	2	84 ± 8	84 ± 8	–1					94 ± 9	94 ± 11	0				
Mean pressure (mmHg)															
RA	0	4 ± 2	4 ± 2	0					8 ± 3	9 ± 4	2				
	1	4 ± 2	4 ± 2	0					8 ± 3	8.1 ± 3	0				
	2	4 ± 2	4 ± 2	0					8 ± 3	8 ± 3	0				
PA															
	0	15 ± 3	15 ± 3	0					37 ± 7	39 ± 9	4	*			
	1	15 ± 3	15 ± 4	0					38 ± 10	36 ± 9	–5				
	2	15 ± 4	16 ± 4	2					37 ± 10	36 ± 10	–3				

Table 1 continued

PC							
	0	8 ± 3	7 ± 3	–11	26 ± 8	27 ± 9	3
	1	8 ± 4	8 ± 3	0	25 ± 8	24 ± 8	–5
	2	9 ± 3	8 ± 3	–9	24 ± 10	23 ± 9	–6
Cardiac index (l/min × m^2)							
	0	3.12 ± 0.62	3.12 ± 0.67	0	6.49 ± 1.82	6.35 ± 1.60	–2
	1	3.31 ± 0.65	3.30 ± 0.57	0	6.26 ± 1.78	6.32 ± 1.73	1
	2	3.23 ± 0.52	3.09 ± 0.48	–4	5.99 ± 1.47	6.11 ± 1.39	2
Syst. vasc. resist. (dyn s × cm^{-5})							
	0	1420 ± 295	1489 ± 396	5	843 ± 266	863 ± 278	2
	1	1278 ± 255	1264 ± 264	–1	820 ± 247	792 ± 206	–3
	2	1364 ± 301	1360 ± 238	0	842 ± 201	817 ± 200	–3

Notation:
RA = right atrial pressure; PA = pulmonary artery pressure; PC = pulmonary capillary pressure; syst. vasc. resist = systemic vascular resistance; chg.% = changes in %, control = 100 %, sign (A) = significance A = intragroup evaluation control vs placebo or 2.5 mg, 5 mg ULFS 49 CL, methods: *t*-test for paired samples, Pitman-Morgan test; sign. (B) = significance B = ANOVA of differences with ordered groups, paired comparisons according to Scheffe. No significance = blank field. The intergroup comparisons and significances are given cross-over in the column significance B.

by **, and $p < 0.001$ by ***. Group 0 (Gr 0) received placebo, group 1 (Gr 1) 2.5 mg ULFS 49 CL, and group 2 (Gr 2) 5 mg ULFS 49 CL.

Results

A total of 114 patients were included in the trial, one of whom did not receive the study medication because he developed unstable angina before administration. Another seven patients had to be excluded from the statistical evaluation, because they did not meet various inclusion criteria. The distribution of evaluated patients revealed a predominance of male patients (n = 92). Their mean age was 58 ± 8 years. The mean age of the female patients (n = 14) was 57 ± 6 years. The mean height of all patients was 171 ± 8 cm and the mean body weight was 75.3 ± 9.7 kg.

Resting heart rate was significantly reduced only by 5 mg ULFS 49 CL ($p < 0.5$), however, exercise heart rate was reduced by 5 % in both active treatment groups ($p < .001$), with no difference between the two groups. There were no significant changes in any of the groups regarding systolic and diastolic blood pressure, pulmonary artery and capillary pressures, right atrial pressure, cardiac index and systemic vascular resistance (Table 1).

Table 2.

	During exercise, last comp. values							
Parameter (dim.)	Gr.	Control	Placebo or ULFS 49 CL	Chg. %	Sign. (A)	Sign. (B)		
						gr. 0	gr. 1	gr. 2
Workload (w × min)	0	649 ± 349	639 ± 346	–2				
	1	538 ± 368	598 ± 346	11	*			
	2	513 ± 280	555 ± 285	8				
Exercise duration								
(s)	0	671 ± 216	667 ± 217	–1				
	1	604 ± 219	659 ± 223	9	*			
	2	593 ± 206	627 ± 192	6				
Time to anginal pain								
(s)	0	457 ± 209	461 ± 201	1				
	1	437 ± 214	488 ± 213	12				
	2	404 ± 197	460 ± 178	14	*			
Time until 1st ST-segment depression								
> = 0.1(s)	0	316 ± 182	350 ± 177	11				
	1	323 ± 184	405 ± 200	25	**			
	2	294 ± 205	358 ± 193	22	*			

Notation:
see Table 1.

Exercise capacity, evaluated in workload (watts × min.) increased significantly ($p < .05$) in the 2.5 mg group by 60 watts × min., but failed, however, to reach the significance level in the 5 mg group with an increase of 42 watts × min (Table 2).

Time until onset of first ST-segment depression of at least 0.1 mv was significantly prolonged by 82 s in the 2.5 mg group ($p < .05$) and by 64 s in the 5 mg group ($p < .01$) (Table 2).

Only treatment with 5 mg ULFS 49 CL significantly prolonged the time until onset of anginal pain by 56 s ($p < .05$), whereas the 51 s improvement in the 2.5 mg group failed to reach the significance level and placebo increased the time by only 4 s (Table 2).

ULFS 49 CL clearly influenced the maximal sum of ST-segment depression. There was a reduction by 29 % ($p < .01$) in the 2.5 mg group and by 22 % ($p < 0.001$) in the 5 mg group, whereas no effect was observed with placebo (Fig. 1).

ULFS 49 CL plasma concentration was assessed from blood sampled 15 min after injection. Mean plasma concentrations measured by HPLC were 35 ± 40 ng/ml in the 2.5 mg group and 60 ± 120 ng/ml in the 5 mg group.

The surface ECG (lead III, V_2, V_4 and V_6) did not show any significant changes in the width of the QRS complex, duration of the P-wave, or PQ duration, neither at rest nor at exercise (data not depicted). Only one adverse event ("feeling one's heart") was reported in the 5 mg group, supporting the good tolerability of ULFS 49 CL.

Summary of results

ULFS 49 CL proved to be efficacious in patients suffering from angina pectoris, the antiischemic effects being more pronounced than the antianginal efficacy. Heart rate was slightly, however, significantly decreased both at rest and exercise. The observed effects after administration of a single dose appear to be independent from the dose.

Discussion

The present study indicates that ULFS 49 CL is able to produce favorable antiischemic effects in patients with coronary artery disease which are comparable to those of established β-blockers. Drug-induced changes in heart rate, however, were three to four times less pronounced (especially during exercise) than could be expected from a β-blocker administered in a therapeutic dose. The apparent lack of significant changes in hemodynamic parameters argues against a reduction of pre- or afterload which could be responsible for this antiischemic effect, as suggested for calcium antagonists or nitrates.

ULFS 49 CL does not influence β adrenoceptors (unpublished data from Dr. Karl Thomae GmbH). Preliminary results from the muscarinic working group at the Kerckhoff Clinic, Bad Nauheim, showed that the K-value of ULFS 49 CL on M_2 cholinoceptors was 15.8 μg/ml (unpublished data). An interaction with muscarinic receptors can be excluded, since the free drug concentration in the two verum-

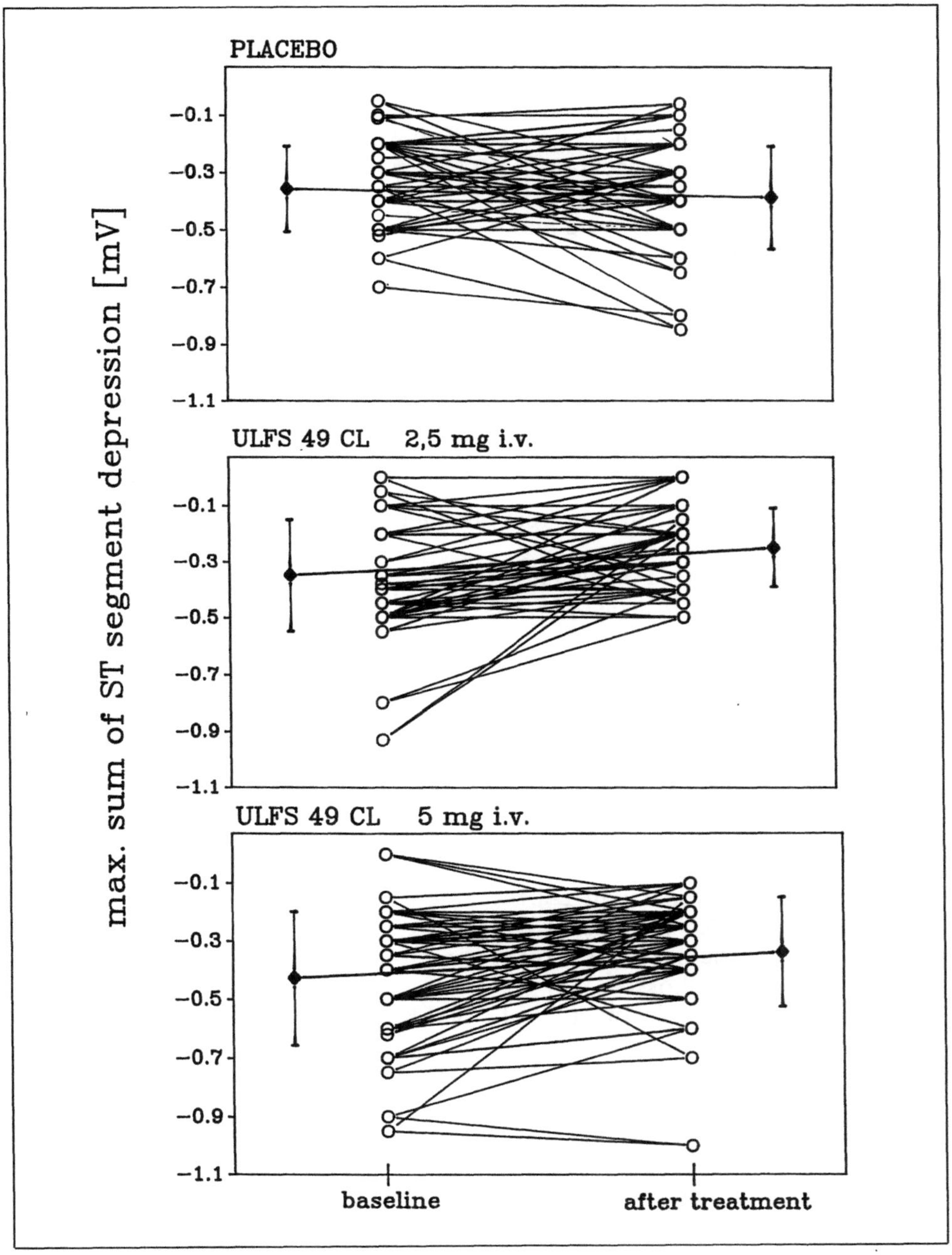

Fig. 1. The maximum sum of ST-segment depression was read from lead III, V2, V4, and V6. The starting points of the lines of the individual patients on the left side are the control values derived at maximum workload without premedication. The endpoints on the right side of the figure were those derived at maximum workload after treatment with either placebo (upper panel), 2.5 mg ULFS 49 CL (middle panel), or 5.0 mg ULFS 49 CL (lower panel). The thick line in each panel connects the means of each group, which are given as ±SD.

treated groups was in the range of 10^{-8} to 10^{-9} g/ml. As the compound is protein-bound to about 90%, an unspecific interaction with muscarinic receptor systems appears to be impossible.

Therefore, the observed reduction of the heart rate is best explained by the known inhibition of the i_f current by ULFS 49 CL. However, it remains unclear whether the marked antiischemic effect of ULFS 49 CL are solely caused by the minor reduction of the heart rate.

The question of the underlying mechanism of action and, in addition, the proof that ULFS 49 CL has benefits over other antianginal medication (i.e., less contraindications, less side effects, no negative effects on lipid and carbohydrate metabolism) are important for the planning of future clinical trials with this agent.

Acknowledgements:

Data reported in this publication were obtained from patients from the following eight trial centers:

1) Kerckhoff-Klinik, Bad Nauheim:
   Prof. Dr. med. Martin Schlepper, Dr. med. H. F. Pitschner, Dr. med. E. Muno, Dr. med. S. Schulte, Dr. med. F. Vens-Cappell.
2) Klinik Mühlenberg, Fachabteilung Angiologie:
   Dr. med. K.-J. Nordmann, Dr. med. W. Grote.
3) Klinikum der Albrecht-Ludwig-Universität, Innere Medizin III/Kardiologie, Freiburg:
   Prof. Dr. med. H. Just, PD Dr. med. Ch. Holubarsch, Dr. med. L. Tierfelder.
4) Klinik Martinsquelle für Herz- und Kreislauf, Abt. Innere Medizin/Kardiologie, Bad Lippspringe
5) Medizinische Universität zu Lübeck, Intensivkardiologie, Lübeck:
   Prof. Dr. med. A. Sheikzadeh, Dr. med. R. Mitusch.
6) Herz- und Kreislaufzentrum Rotenburg, Rotenburg a.d. Fulda:
   Prof. Dr. med. F. Loskot..
7) Schüchtermann Klinik, Innere Abt., Bad Rothenfelde:
   Dr. med. M. Karoff.
8) Kurklinik Königsfeld der LVA Westfalen, Ennepetal-Milspe:
   Dr. med. M. Karoff.

We thank all our colleagues for their engagement and work which were the basis for this publication. The trial was financially supported by Dr. Karl Thomae GmbH, Chemisch-Pharmazeutische Fabrik, Biberach an der Riß.

References

1. Lillie C, Kobinger W (1986) Investigations into the bradycardic effects of ULFS 49 CL (1,3,4,5-tetrahydro-7,8-dimethoxy-3-3-(3-k((2-(3,4-dimethoxyphenyl))ethyl) methylimino-propyl)-2H-3-benzazepin-2-on-hydrochloride) in isolated guinea pig atria. J Cardiovasc Pharmacol 8: 791–797.

2. Krumpl G, Schneider W, Raberger G (1986) Can exercise-induced regional contractile dysfunction be prevented by selective bradycardic agents? Naunyn-Schmiedebergs Arch Pharmacol 334: 540–543.
3. Le CG (1987) On testing a trend in means in oneway layout. Biometrical Journal 29/2: 173–180.
4. Morrison DF (Multivariate statistical methods. International Student Edition. McGraw-Hill International Book Company. Auckland Bogota Guatema Hamburg Johannesburg Lisbon London Madrid Mexico New Delhi Panama Paris San Juan Sao Paulo Singapore Sydney Tokyo. 2. Edition, 4th print 1982.

Authors' address:
Dr. H. F. Pitschner
Kerckhoff-Klinik
Max-Planck-Gesellschaft
Benekestraße 2
6350 Bad Nauheim

Efficacy and duration of action of three doses of Zatebradine (ULFS 49 CL) in patients with chronic angina pectoris compared to placebo

W. Baiker[1], E. v. Czako[2], M. Keck[3] and G. Nehmiz[4]

[1] Department of Medicine, Cardiology, Dr. Karl Thomae GmbH, Biberach, FRG; [2] Salzetalklinik der LVA Westfalen, Bad Sulzuflen, FRG; [3] Fachklinik für Herz- und Kreislaufkrankheiten der LVA, Bad Münster am Stein, FRG; [4] Department of Medicine, Biometry, Dr. Karl Thomae GmbH, Biberach, FRG

Introduction

Zatebradine (ULFS 49 CL) is a member of a new class of drugs, the so-called sinus node inhibitors that specifically reduce the spontaneous rate of depolarization of the pacemaker cells in the sino-atrial node [5, 6], leading to a decrease in heart rate.

This results in a reduction of myocardial oxygen demand. Moreover, the prolongation of diastole together with unaltered perfusion pressure may improved oxygen supply to the myocardium.

One study in which zatebradine was administered intravenously as a single dose demonstrated already marked acute antiischemic and antianginal efficacy [3].

The present study was undertaken to evaluate the oral efficacy and the dose relationship of zatebradine in patients with chronic stable angina pectoris.

Patients and methods

Patients

A total of 182 patients were enrolled into the placebo run-in period of this clinical trial by nine centers. Of these, 174 patients qualified for the double-blind treatment period.

To be admitted to the study, patients had to have a history of exertional angina pectoris, which had to be stable for at least 3 months. Angina had to be inducible by a baseline bicycle ergometry test, and associated with ST-segment depression of at least 1 mm. Also, patients had to be in sinus rhythm and experience at least three anginal attacks per week under standard treatment. The age range was 40–75 years, both men and postmenopausal women being eligible.

Cardiovascular drugs other than sublingual nitrates for relief of anginal attacks had to be withdrawn at least 3 days before entry in the study. Verbal or written informed consent was obtained. Major exclusion criteria were unstable angina, myocardial infarction within the preceding 3 months, uncontrolled hypertension, and any significant systemic disease.

Exercise testing

Maximum symptom-limited exercise tests were performed on a bicycle in sitting position. The starting load was determined individually by a test carried out after 1 week of placebo run-in. The initial load in this was 25 W, followed by incremental steps of 25 W every 3 minutes.

Subsequent tests were started with two loadsteps below the maximally reached load, and were increased by 25 W every 3 min. Blood pressure was recorded according to the method of Riva-Rocci at the end of each load step, at the end of the ergometry, and 6 min after stop of exercise. Simultaneously, heart rate was recorded and averaged from the last 20 cycles of the ECG-strip.

Total exercise time, time to onset of angina, and time to 1-mm ST-segment depression, 80 msec after the J-point, as well as ST-segment depression at the end of each exercise step were recorded.

Total work was calculated by multiplying the loadstep reached by total exercise duration. The exercise tests were performed 2 hours (day 2, day 13) and 10 hours (day 1, day 14) after drug administration.

Anginal attacks and consumption of sublingual nitrates

Patients kept diaries to record the number of daily anginal attacks and number of consumed sublingual nitrates. For comparison the last week of the placebo run-in period and the last week of the double-blind period were used.

Study drug and concomitant medication

All study medication was provided in identical capsules containing placebo, 1.25 mg, 2.5 mg or 5 mg zatebradine (ULFS 49 CL). All study medication was taken in a bid regimen. All cardiovascular medication, except sublingual nitrates for relief of anginal attacks were withdrawn. All other medication had to be kept constant throughout the trial whenever possible.

Drug safety

Adverse events, whether or not considered to be drug-related were recorded, if reported spontaneously or elicited by a general question as to the patient's health. Additionally, standard hematological and serum biochemistry tests were performed at baseline and after the trial.

Randomization

According to a randomization list, patients were chronologically allocated to one of the four treatment groups.

Statistical methods

Changes of qualitative data were compared with the one-sample Wilcoxon-test (exact) and the Kruskal-Wallis test (asymptotic). Quantitative data were tested by one-way analysis of variance with ordered groups and Scheffe's method. Data are expressed as mean ± SD.

Study design (Fig. 1)

After screening for inclusion and exclusion criteria, eligible patients from whom informed consent was obtained had their previous antianginal medication withdrawn for at least 3 days. Then they were treated with placebo capsules for 2 weeks (run-in period). Diaries were issued for documentation of anginal attacks and consumption of sublingual nitrates. Patients were instructed not to use nitrates prophylactically. After 1 week, the first symptom-limited exercise test was performed to determine the starting load for all subsequent tests. These were performed 10 hours p.a. and 2 hours p.a. to determine baseline values. A blood sample was drawn for safety laboratory variables and double-blind therapy was

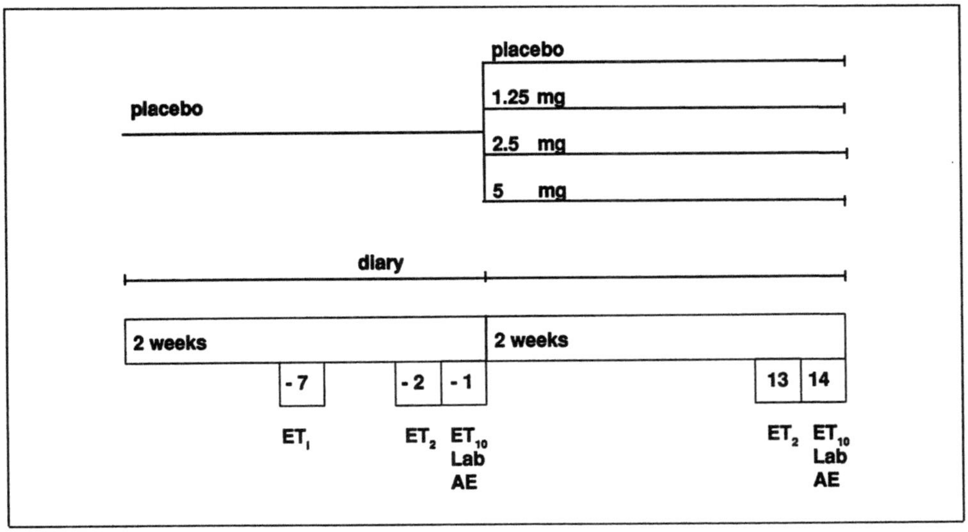

Fig. 1. Study design:
ET_1 = excercise test to determine starting load
ET_2 = exercise test 2 h p. a.
ET_{10} = exercise test 10 h p. a.
Lab = routine hematology and clinical chemistry
AE = documentation of adverse events

initiated for 2 weeks. End-of-treatment exercise tests were performed on day 13 (2 hours p.a.) and day 14 (10 hours p.a.). Adverse events were reported and another blood sample was taken.

Results

Among the 182 patients enrolled in the study, eight did not qualify for the double-blind period (two patients) or dropped out due to worsening of angina (six patients). Hence, 174 patients entered the double-blind treatment phase and received placebo (46 patients), 1.25 mg (43 patients), 2.5 mg (40 patients) or 5 mg (45 patients) zatebradine, twice daily.

A total of seven patients were excluded from the efficacy analysis, because they did not comply with the study protocol; five discontinued due to increase in anginal attacks (placebo, n = 2), nausea (1.25 mg, n = 1), transfer to planned PTCA (2.5 mg, n = 1), and dizziness (5 mg, n = 1). The remaining 162 patients were evaluated for efficacy. All 174 entering the double-blind period were evaluated for safety.

Exercise testing

The results of analysis of major exercise test variables are summarized in Table 1. Total exercise work was considered the primary endpoint. Total work increased from 636 ± 317 W minutes on placebo to 685 ± 429 W minutes (n.s.), from 588 ± 286 on 1.25 mg zatebradine to 666 ± 330 W minutes ($p < 0.01$), from 580 ± 291 W minutes on 2.5 mg to 725 ± 346 W minutes ($p < 0.001$), and from 562 ± 259 W minutes on 5 mg to 811 ± 318 W minutes ($p < 0.001$) 2 hours after administration of the trial drug. The dose trend was statistically significant $p < 0.001$.

10 hours after administration, total exercise work was increased by 40 ± 219 W minutes on placebo (n.s.), by 56 ± 155 W minutes on 1.25 mg ($p < 0.05$), by 130 ± 180 W minutes on 2.5 mg ($p < 0.001$) and by 189 ± 242 W minutes on 5 mg zatebradine bid ($p < 0.001$) with a statistically significant dose trend with $p < 0.001$ (Fig. 2).

Table 1. Changes of major exercise parameters after 2 weeks of treatment with study drug administered twice daily.

	Placebo	1.25 mg	2.5 mg	5 mg	Dose trend
Workload					
2 h p. a. [W min]	49 ± 204	78 ± 157	145 ± 179	249 ± 248	$p < 0.001$
10 h p. a. [W min]	40 ± 219	56 ± 155	130 ± 180	189 ± 242	$p < 0.001$
Exercise duration					
2 h p. a. [sec]	14 ± 107	37 ± 105	79 ± 94	131 ± 127	$p < 0.001$
10 h p. a. [sec]	19 ± 123	25 ± 86	70 ± 102	104 ± 120	$p < 0.001$
Time to 1-mm ST ↓					
2 h p. a. [sec]	1 ± 101	33 ± 80	90 ± 98	100 ± 82	$p < 0.001$
10 h p. a. [sec]	9 ± 90	38 ± 103	52 ± 106	56 ± 98	$p < 0.05$

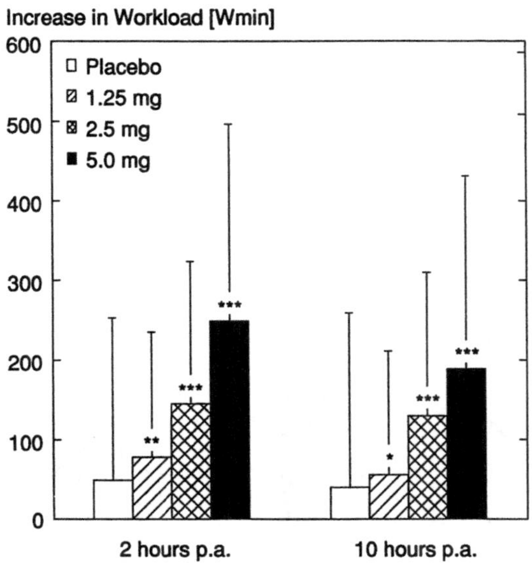

Fig. 2. Increase in exercise workload after 2 weeks treatment. Dose trend statistically significant at both timepoints $p < .001$.

Using Scheffe's method for pairwise comparison, 5 mg total exercise work with zatebradine was significantly different from placebo ($p < 0.05$) and from 1.25 mg zatebradine ($p < 0.05$). All other possible comparisons did not differ statistically.

The change in time to 1-mm ST-segment depression was 1 ± 101 seconds on placebo (n.s.), 33 ± 80 s. on 1.25 mg ($p < 0.05$), 90 ± 98 s on 2.5 mg ($p < 0.001$), and 100 ± 82 s on 5 mg ($p < 0.001$) with a significant dose trend ($p < 0.001$). 10 hours after administration the anti-ischemic effect of zatebradine was maintained in all three doses (Fig. 3).

When changes in exercise duration are expressed in percent, placebo increased exercise time by 3% (n.s.) 2 h p.a. and by 4% (n.s.) 10 h.p.a. 1.25 mg zatebradine improved exercise time by 8% ($p < 0.05$) and 5% ($p < 0.05$), respectively. 2.5 mg showed an increase of 16% ($p < 0.001$) and 14% ($p < 0.001$), respectively, whereas 5 mg zatebradine administered twice daily for 2 weeks increased total exercise duration by 29% ($p < 0.001$) and 23%, respectively (Fig. 4).

Heart rate reduction at rest and at the last common loadstep is shown in Table 2, both for the exercise tests at 2 hours and at 10 hours post administration. There are statistically significant dose trends at both timepoints, although the comparison to baseline was not always significant.

Anginal attacks and sublingual nitrate consumption

The number of anginal attacks and of sublingual nitrates were reduced in all four treatment groups with significant dose trends, both for reduction in anginal attacks ($p < 0.001$) and consumption of short-acting nitrates ($p < 0.01$) (Table 3).

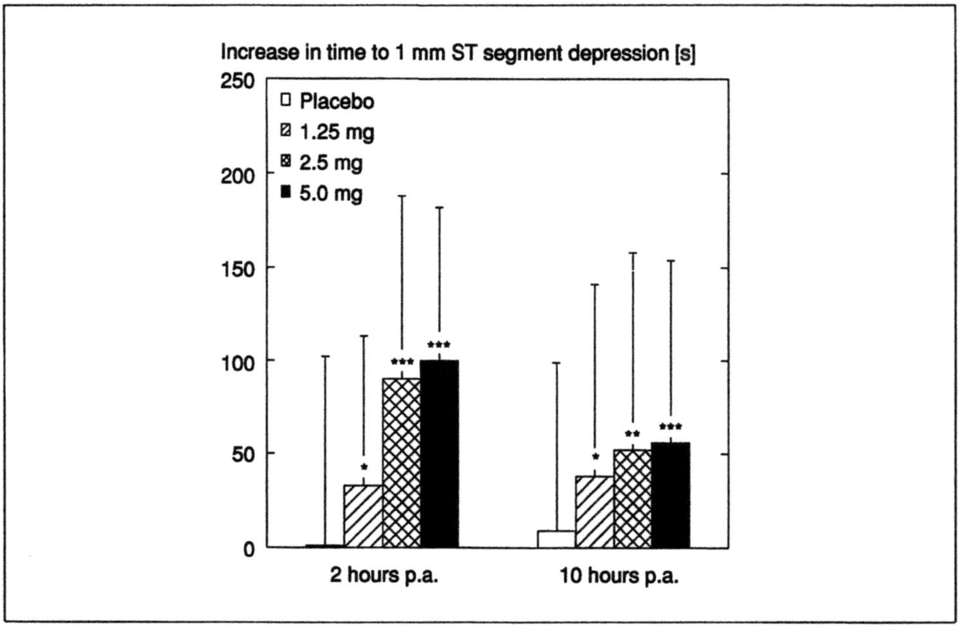

Fig. 3. Increase in time to 1 mm ST-segment depression after 2 weeks treatment. Dose trend statistically significant 2 h p.a. $p < .001$; 10 h p.a. $p < .05$.

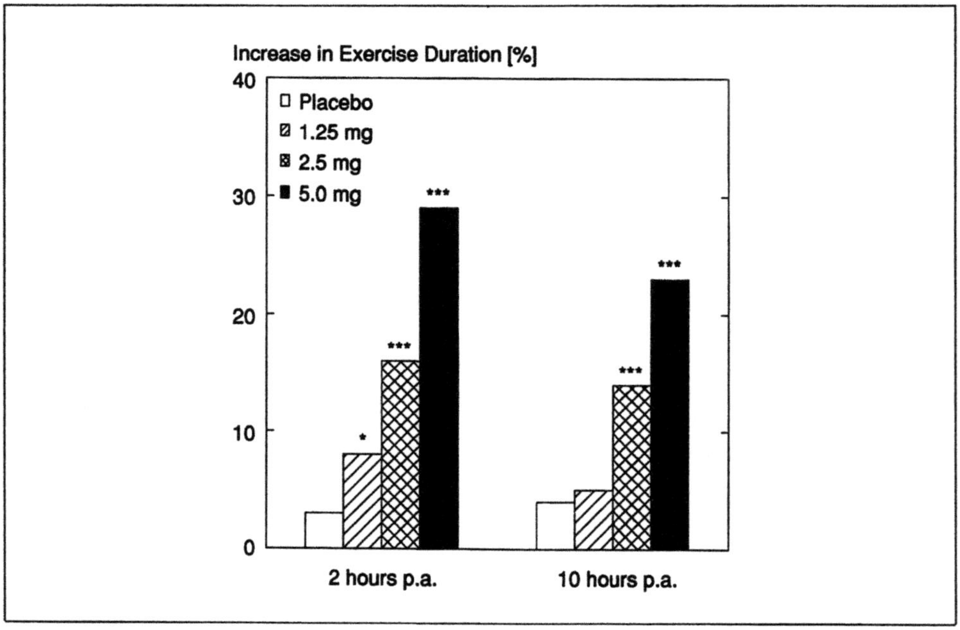

Fig. 4. Change in exercise duration after 2 weeks treatment. Dose trend statistically significant at both timepoints $p < .001$.

Table 2. Reduction in heart rate at rest and at exercise (last common loadstep) after 2 weeks of treatment with study drug administered twice daily.

	Placebo	1.25 mg	2.5 mg	5 mg	Dose trend
Heart rate at rest					
2 h p. a.	− 3 ± 10	− 2 ± 9	− 3 ± 8	− 8 ± 10	$p < 0.05$
10 h p. a.	0 ± 8	− 2 ± 7	− 1 ± 8	− 5 ± 9	$p < 0.05$
Heart rate at exercise					
2 h p. a.	− 5 ± 13	− 6 ± 11	− 8 ± 15	− 12 ± 13	$p < 0.01$
10 h p. a.	− 2 ± 13	− 4 ± 11	− 6 ± 10	− 9 ± 12	$p < 0.01$

Table 3. Reduction in number of anginal attacks and number of s.l. nitrates consumed after 2 weeks treatment with study drug administered twice daily.

	Placebo	1.25 mg	2.5 mg	5 mg	Dose trend
Anginal attacks per week	− 1.7 ± 5.3	− 3.3 ± 4.9	− 3.4 ± 5.9	− 4.2 ± 4.8	$p < 0.001$
Nitrate consumption per week	− 1.7 ± 6.2	− 4.3 ± 6.2	− 3.8 ± 9.4	− 5.3 ± 7.6	$p < 0.01$

Adverse events on treatment and laboratory

The adverse events which occurred during the double-blind treatment phase are shown in Table 4 according to their system-organ classes.

There was no accummulation of any of the adverse events, nor was there a dose trend in their frequency.

Table 4. Adverse events during double-blind treatment according to WHO System-Organ-Classes.

System-Organ-Class	Placebo	1.25 mg	2.5 mg	5 mg
Skin and appendage disorders	1	1	0	0
Centr. & periph. nervous syst. disorders	1	1	1	1
Psychiatric disorders	0	0	0	1
Gastrointestinal disorders	2	5	1	0
Cardiovascular disorders, general	0	1	1	0
Myo-, endo-, pericardial & valve disorders	1	0	0	0
Heart rate and rhythm disorders	0	2	0	1
Respiratory system disorders	0	0	0	2
Urinary system disorders	1	0	0	1
Body as a whole	1	3	0	4
Without adverse events	40	36	37	38
Total patients treated	46	43	40	45

All laboratory parameters remained within the normal biological range. There were some statistically significant changes in all groups, which were, however, not clinically relevant and not dose-dependent.

Discussion

Data on the effect of zatebradine on exercise performance in patients with angina pectoris which have been published to date are limited to one study, in which the effects of 5 mg and 10 mg zatebradine, given intravenously, were compared to placebo [3]. In this acute study, 5 mg zatebradine acutely prolonged exercise duration by 22 %, 10 mg prolonged it by 27 %, and placebo by 9 %. These effects were maintained during a subchronic treatment period of 2 weeks.

A reduction in heart rate is the mechanism supposedly [3] responsible for the efficacy of the drug. The relatively small reduction in heart rate compared to the marked antianginal and anti-ischemic efficacy is disturbing, however, in pigs it could be demonstrated that zatebradine almost exclusively prolongs diastole, leaving the systolic time unchanged [7].

Alinidine, another drug that specifically reduces heart rate, was compared to propranolol, a β-adrenoceptor antagonist, in order to investigate the relationship between heart rate and diastolic period [2]. It could be demonstrated that alinidine increased the diastolic period to a greater extent than did the β-blocker. In another trial, alinidine was compared to metoprolol [1]. Despite a much smaller reduction in heart rate compared to metoprolol, alinidine improved exercise tolerance similar to the β-blocker. These results indicate that besides the selective reduction of heart rate, a prolongation of diastole may be responsible for the antianginal efficacy of heart-rate reducing agents (sinus node inhibitors) such as alinidine and zatebradine.

Moreover, a recent study performed in an animal model of ischemia [4] indicates that the myocardial blood flow per beat is an important predictor of ischemia. Since zatebradine does not reduce blood pressure, the myocardial blood flow per beat is markedly improved and may be an explanation for the efficacy in patients with chronic stable angina pectoris.

Conclusion

2.5 mg and 5 mg zatebradine administered twice daily for 2 weeks revealed marked antianginal and anti-ischemic efficacy which was maintained for at least 10 h after administration. With respect to the 10 hours post administration data, the improvement with the 1.25 mg dose is probably not clinically significant. Therefore, 2.5 mg may be considered as the minimally effective dose. Zatebradine was well tolerated and did not demonstrate a dose trend in any of the adverse events reported.

These data suggest that zatebradine may be useful to treat patients with chronic stable angina pectoris effectively and safely.

Summary

Zatebradine (ULFS 49 CL), a new antianginal agent (1.25 mg, 2.5 mg, 5 mg bid) was compared in three doses to placebo for subchronic treatment of patients with chronic stable angina pectoris.

After wash-out and placebo run-in, 174 patients were randomly and double-blindly allocated to one of the four treatment groups. Two symptom-limited exercise tests (2 h and 10 h p.a.) were performed at the end of the placebo run-in period, and after 2 weeks of double-blind treatment. Diaries were kept by the patients throughout the trial in order to record anginal attacks and s.l. nitrate consumption.

There was a clear and dose-dependent improvement in total exercise tolerance and exercise time to onset of angina and 1-mm ST-segment depression. This effect was also demonstrable 10 h after application for 2.5 mg and 5 mg zatebradine bid. Generally, zatebradine was well tolerated and the incidence of adverse events did not differ from placebo.

Acknowledgement

The following trial centers participated in this clinical study: H. Bouzo, Augsburg; E. v. Czako, Bad Salzuflen; M. Hilbert, Bredstedt, U. Hildebrandt, Prien; F. Jentzen, Kiel; M. Keck, Bad Münster; G. Müller, Königstein; E. Volger, Bad Wörishofen and N. Warlo, Kriftel.

We thank Mrs. H. Carstanjen for documentation and assistance in the preparation of the statistical evaluation.

References

1. Balakumaran K, Jovanovic A, Fels Ph. W, van Es GA, Bokslag M, Lubsen J, Hugenholtz PG (1987) AT 567 (alinidine) in stable angina: a comparison with metoprolol. Eur Heart J 8 (Suppl L) 153–157.
2. Ferro G, Spinelli L, Duilio C, Spadafora M, Cinquegrana G, Condorelli M (1990) Alinidine in chronic stable angina: The effect on diastolic perfusion time. Cardiology 77: 287–294.
3. Hauf DF, Rose P. Schnellbacher K. Roskamm H (1990) Effect of ULFS 49 CL in patients with stable angina pectoris. Z Kardiol 79 (Suppl 1): Abstr P556.
4. Indolfi C, C, Guth BD, Miura T, Miyazaki S, Schulz R, Ross J Jr. (1989) Mechanism of improved ischemic regional dysfunction by bradycardia; Studies on ULFS 49 in swine. Circulation 80 No. 4: 983–993.
5. Lillie C, Kobinger W (1986) Investigations into the bradycardic efects of ULFS 49 CL in isolated guinea pig atria. J Cardiovasc Pharmacol 8: 791–797
6. Van Ginneken ACG, Bouman LN, Jongsma HJ, Duivenvoorden JJ, Opthof T, Giler WR (1987) Alinidine as a model of the mode of action of specific bradycardic agents on SA node activity. Eur Heart J 8 (Suppl L): 25–33.
7. Van Woerkens LJ, van der Giessen WJ, Verdouw PD (1991) The selective bradycardic effects of ULFS 49 do not adversely affect left ventricular function in conscious pigs with chronic coronary artery occlusion. Cardiovasc Drugs Ther 5: 000–000 submitted for publication.

Authors' address:
W. Baiker
Associate Director, Clinical Research
Boehringer Ingelheim Pharmaceuticals Inc.
90 East Ridge
Ridgefield, CT 06877

GPSR Compliance

The European Union's (EU) General Product Safety Regulation (GPSR) is a set of rules that requires consumer products to be safe and our obligations to ensure this.

If you have any concerns about our products, you can contact us on ProductSafety@springernature.com

In case Publisher is established outside the EU, the EU authorized representative is:

Springer Nature Customer Service Center GmbH
Europaplatz 3
69115 Heidelberg, Germany

Batch number: 10577969

Printed by Printforce, the Netherlands